"Got a body? Wanna love God? Then [...] everyone's book. Here is the terrific news Rob Moll g[...] smartest sources: not just that we have bodies, but we *are* bodies, and we've been marvelously wired and equipped to love God and serve our neighbor with and through these wondrous creations. Who does not need to hear this—our bodies are not a curse but a gift. Thank you, Mr. Moll."

Leslie Leyland Fields, author and contributing editor, *Christianity Today*

"It's always exciting a read to a book whose core insight makes such intuitive sense but whose implications have gone underexplored. Rob Moll's work is engrossing and informative, and you can act on it right away. And at the book's heart is a really encouraging message grounded in solid research: when you look at your body closely, you'll find out that you're designed to be who you really want to be."

Patton Dodd, editor in chief, OnFaith

"This book goes behind the genetic curtain to show the intricate and exceptional design within our bodies to provide groundbreaking point—we're not only called to worship, but beautifully wired to do so."

Brian Orme, editor, *Outreach* magazine

"Rob Moll uses the best in neuroscience to illuminate what biblical scholars have been telling us about God's purpose for embodied existence. We are not alien souls locked in inhospitable bodies, but we were made to be spiritual through our flesh and bone. This is an important book for couples who care about each other's bodies to read together."

David Neff, former editor in chief, *Christianity Today*

"Marshaling cutting-edge neuroscience, theological acumen and deft storytelling, this book of Rob Moll's invites us to honor the way the Creator God formed us in the *imago Dei*: as integrated wholes—body, mind and spirit all one. We have much to learn from Moll's work—may it lead many into deeper awe and wonder at the great goodness of the incarnate God, and the flourishing life we are invited into."

Michael Yankoski, author of *Under the Overpass* and *The Sacred Year*

"One of the most mysterious yet inspirational statements in Scripture is that we are created in the image of God. There's a purpose behind human existence, and it involves every one of us, and all aspects of us. Somehow it connects us with God. If that's true, then we'd expect there to be evidence that we are made in a way that can reflect the very capacities of God—to love, to create, etc. Rob Moll has done a great service by gathering that evidence in one place. *What Your Body Knows About God* is a marvelous testimony to how science and Scripture are complementary rather than contradictory."

John Kilner, Forman Chair of Christian Ethics and Theology, Trinity International University

"Every day it seems we read about new scientific studies that reveal fascinating insights into the operation of the human mind and body. But as Christians we sometimes wonder whether these studies challenge our assumptions from the Bible. Will they attempt to explain away the power of prayer? The possibility of spiritual transformation? The need for intimate human community? My friend Rob Moll has helped us by pulling together the latest research and showing how it fits with Christian teaching on how we grow in love of God and each other. I hope you learn as much as I did about God's wonderful plan of creation."

Collin Hansen, editorial director, The Gospel Coalition, and author of *Young, Restless, Reformed: A Journalist's Journey with the New Calvinists*

"Rob Moll must have paid better attention in science class than most of us did. The result is a book I literally could not stop referencing in my preaching. Science is seeing what faith has long known—that discipleship can make us more sane, healthy, human."

Jason Byassee, senior pastor, Boone United Methodist Church, North Carolina; fellow in theology and leadership, Duke Divinity School, and author of *Discerning the Body*

"In *What Your Body Knows About God*, Rob Moll has successfully brought together research, personal experience and biblical analysis to show how our bodies were made to engage with the Almighty God. You will be hard pressed to find another book with such high-level research, while remaining a high-quality read. Pastors, parishioners and nonbelievers will all benefit from this foundational work in understanding the intersection between humanity and divinity."

Tyler Braun, pastor, author of *Why Holiness Matters*

"Human biology may have lulled me to sleep in college, but *What Your Body Knows About God* kept me riveted and up way too late as Moll explores the fascinating connections between the physical and spiritual, the material and the mystical. A must-read!"

Caryn Rivadeneira, author of *Broke*; co-host and producer, *Midday Connection*, Moody Radio

"In Rob Moll's second book, he brings his considerable skill, insight and winsome curiosity to bear on the connection between the body, the brain and spiritual practice. This latest effort will encourage a new level of interest among Christians in the relationship between the flesh and the spirit. I warmly recommend it to readers."

Hunter Baker, dean of instruction, Union University, and author of *The End of Secularism*

"*What Your Body Knows About God* evokes wonder and worship as Moll skillfully guides the reader through the astonishing complexity of bodies and minds and how human beings relate to one another—and to God. A must-read for those curious about spirituality and science, and the relationship between the two."

Rachel Marie Stone, author of *Eat With Joy: Redeeming God's Gift of Food*

"Moll's knack for presenting thought-provoking material in an easy-going conversational style makes *What Your Body Knows About God* a pleasure to read. Although replete with scientific information, discussions such as the 'neurological costs' of worship as performance and the transformative benefits of multisensory liturgy leave little doubt that Moll's concern is practical, not theoretical. As such, it is a must-read for pastors, ministers, small group leaders and anyone else concerned with the transformation of people."

Miles S. Mullin II, associate professor of church history, Southwestern Baptist Theological Seminary

WHAT YOUR BODY KNOWS ABOUT GOD

HOW WE ARE DESIGNED TO CONNECT, SERVE AND THRIVE

ROB MOLL

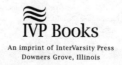

IVP Books

An imprint of InterVarsity Press
Downers Grove, Illinois

InterVarsity Press
P.O. Box 1400, Downers Grove, IL 60515-1426
World Wide Web: www.ivpress.com
Email: email@ivpress.com

*InterVarsity Press® is the book-publishing division of InterVarsity Christian Fellowship/USA®, a
movement of students and faculty active on campus at hundreds of universities, colleges and schools
of nursing in the United States of America, and a member movement of the International Fellowship
of Evangelical Students. For information about local and regional activities, visit intervarsity.org.*

*All Scripture quotations, unless otherwise indicated, are taken from THE HOLY BIBLE, NEW
INTERNATIONAL VERSION®, NIV® Copyright © 1973, 1978, 1984, 2011 by Biblica, Inc.™ Used
by permission. All rights reserved worldwide.*

*While all stories in this book are true, some names and identifying information in this book have
been changed to protect the privacy of the individuals involved.*

Cover design: Cindy Kiple
Interior design: Beth McGill
Images: © vadimmmus/iStockphoto
Author photo: Alisa Clark

ISBN 978-0-8308-3677-2 (print)
ISBN 978-0-8308-9670-7 (digital)

Printed in the United States of America ♾

 *As a member of the Green Press Initiative, InterVarsity Press is committed to
protecting the environment and to the responsible use of natural resources. To learn
more, visit greenpressinitiative.org.*

Library of Congress Cataloging-in-Publication Data

Moll, Rob, 1977-
  What your body knows about God : how we are designed to connect,
serve, and thrive / Rob Moll.
    pages cm
  Includes bibliographical references.
  ISBN 978-0-8308-3677-2 (pbk. : alk. paper)
  1. Human body—Religious aspects—Christianity. 2. Brain—Religious
aspects—Christianity. 3. Spiritual life—Christianity. 4.
Spirituality—Christianity. 5. Christian life. I. Title.
  BT741.3.M65 2014
  233'.5—dc23

                                                      2014024732

P	20	19	18	17	16	15	14	13	12	11	10	9	8	7	6	5	4	3	2	1
Y	31	30	29	28	27	26	25	24	23	22	21	20	19	18	17	16	15	14

To my junior high and high school youth group leaders,
who taught me to pray:

Dad, Daniel, Dean, James, Jeff, John,
Kirk, Marty, Peter and Peter

CONTENTS

FOREWORD

IN PSALM 139 DAVID SINGS of the wonder of the God who "knit [him] together in his mother's womb." It is a song about being completely known by the God from whom there is no escape. Neither heaven nor Sheol nor darkness itself is able to hide David from the God who knows every word before it is on his tongue. One translation reads that for David such knowledge is "too wonderful" (v. 6). If you yourself have never experienced something that is indeed "too wonderful," David would say you have never really seen the work of the God who created our "innermost parts."

Almost at the center of the psalm, David breaks into praise:

> I will praise You
> because I have been remarkably and wonderfully made.
>> (v. 14 HCSB)

Beyond God's inescapability, David worships him for his exquisite creation of David himself. If only the psalmist had used his extraordinary gift of language to list for us the details he found so remarkable. But sadly, he only sings something about his bones, which, like everything else, could not be hidden from God's relentless gaze. (It's okay to be frustrated by the occasional lack of information in the Bible; see Jn 20:20; 21:25.)

If David was right in being amazed so many centuries ago, imagine the songs he might compose today in light of the abundant discoveries that have been made regarding the human body. Perhaps there is a disproportionate lack of awe in those of us who have made it our business, or at least our hobby, to study God's creation and seek to respond appropriately.

Unquestionably at the top of the list of the wonders of God's creation is the human brain. For too long, ever since the beginning of the computer age, it has been viewed as a pale biological copy of a digital processor. We speak of our "hard drive being full" or the need to "reboot" with a cup of coffee. But in the last few decades that allusion has been decimated, as researchers have discovered in more detail how "remarkably and wonderfully made" is the cantaloupe-sized mystery between our ears.

The latest and best estimate for the memory capacity of the human brain is 256 billion gigabytes. Its computing speed and ability to multitask are virtually unmeasurable. Its ability to rewire itself after a devastating injury (referred to as *plasticity*) has only recently begun to be fully appreciated. When was the last time you dropped your laptop only to discover later that it had repaired itself?

It might just be enough to meditate on the breathtaking complexity and mystery of this one small neurological portion of the vast creation of the God who is inescapable. But to begin to discern the ultimate purpose behind that magnificent design would surely be "too wonderful." And that is just what this book is about. Here are just a few fascinating new facts, provided by current researchers, which in themselves would be interesting enough to read, but Rob Moll has connected design with purpose in what I hope may be just the first of many more such books.

Focusing largely on neurological discoveries, Rob unpacks the purpose behind the design: that one facet of our neurological makeup aids in our ability to empathize, that another by design resonates with the need of our neighbor.

Having read the book, perhaps for the first time I can say that I have begun to appreciate how truly remarkably and wonderfully made we are. That appreciation becomes praise when I look back to the One who knit us together in the inescapable darkness of our mother's womb, creating us for his pleasure with the very real innate potential to truly love our neighbors as ourselves.

Michael Card

Introduction

CREATED FOR COMMUNION

WHEN I WAS A BOY, MY FATHER TAUGHT ME that the way things are built matters. Dad worked in a mold manufacturing shop. He built molds into which hot plastic would be injected to form toys, cups, peanut butter jars, and intricate and precise medical technology.

Dad's workbench at the shop was always strewn with blueprints, and as a child I marveled at how he was able to make sense of the confusing array of lines and instructions and drawings. He read them and then cut, ground and polished blocks of steel until they could be used to make delicate IV drips or the dashboards of trucks.

Dad ran his shop and knew more about steel and plastic products than I could fathom. He could explain how the salad-dressing cap was designed or why a cheap trash can wouldn't survive a year's worth of dragging to the curb. But he only occasionally got to see one of his designs at work, to see the full breadth of purpose for the item he had labored over in blueprints and steel shavings. One of those times was when my brother broke his nose.

After my brother got hit in the face by a basketball, it wasn't obvious at first that he had broken his nose. But after the swelling had gone down a week later, his crooked nose made it obvious—he had to have it broken again in order to be set correctly. We sat together in the hospital room as he recovered, my brother more than a bit traumatized for having his nose broken a second time in a matter of weeks. But Dad? Dad was like a kid on Christmas morning. For the first time, Dad was getting to see the IV drip, syringes and hoses that he had spent several years making.

Dad was beside himself with excitement. He peppered the nurses with questions about how the parts worked together. Did they work well? Did they have problems with the components? How did the confusing aspects of the design help the whole apparatus to function as it should? The design required some unusual manufacturing on his part that had never made sense to him.

"So that's why we had to build it like that!" he exclaimed as we walked out to the parking garage that night to head home. After years of precision-grinding steel, studying blueprints and building parts, my dad was able to understand fully the reasons for the design that he had built.

Spirit and Flesh

In our everyday lives, we too find it helpful to understand how things work. We read WebMD to check out whether our symptoms suggest the flu. We watch YouTube tutorials on how to knit, how to carve a turkey or why our car's engine makes a funny noise when we turn the ignition key. It helps to know how things work. But in our spiritual lives, that kind of knowledge isn't simply helpful. It can be life changing.

The Gospel of John tells us that we are born of flesh and the Spirit (Jn 3:6). But what does that mean? How does it work? Often we only have vague ideas about how our spiritual lives interact with our physical ones. We go to church, we pray, we read spiritual books, we worship, and then, somehow, we are made more like Jesus. We emphasize belief and worldview, as if knowing the right things will always lead us to do the right things. And when all goes according to plan, we may experience God or have a powerful moment of transformation. We say we "feel" God's presence, as though it's something palpable. If it is, how can that be? We're not sure exactly what has made that experience possible.

In many ways we are trying to build a Christian life without fully understanding how all the pieces work together. Prayer, Bible reading and church attendance all can bring us closer to God. We trust this with sure faith. But until recently we have known little about how our spirit and flesh are connected—*how* God has formed our bodies such that those activities change us down to our very cells to better commune with him.

For example, we are all taught to pray; we pray before meals, before bed or during devotional time. But how we pray can have very physical effects. Shorter prayers in which we make requests to God—the kind many of us are most familiar with—go undetected by a brain scan. This doesn't mean they don't work or they are not valuable. But it may encourage you toward deeper, longer prayer when you learn that twelve minutes of attentive and focused prayer every day for eight weeks changes the brain significantly enough to be measured in a brain scan.[1] Not only that, but it strengthens areas of the brain involved in social interaction, increasing our sense of compassion and making us more sensitive to other people. It also reduces stress, bringing another measurable physical effect—lower blood pressure. Prayer in this deeper, more attentive way also strengthens the part of the brain that helps us override our emotional and irrational urges. Prayer that seeks communion with God actually makes us more thoughtful and rational, enhances our

sense of peace and well-being, and makes us more compassionate
and responsive to the needs of other people.

Spirit and flesh, it turns out, are intimately intertwined. And
understanding how things work—how our bodies are designed to
commune with God—can enhance our faith and give us a fuller
picture of God's work in the world and in our lives.

Designed for Communion

Today, scientists are suggesting that the brain is designed for spiritual experience. In recent years, a group of neuroscientists have
been studying brain systems that enable people to have spiritual
experiences. As they have traced the lines of the brain in worship
and meditation, these scientists have discovered that the spiritual
circuit that gets exercise in prayer or in church has all kinds of
positive effects. It's as though God created our bodies to live to their
fullest when we love him and love our neighbors as ourselves. This
is what our bodies are *built to do*.

These scientists make no claim that the brain is experiencing
something outside of itself, that a spiritual experience is actually an
encounter with God. "Theoretically, if God wanted to communicate
with us, He, She, or It would create a biology that allows us to communicate. So it makes sense that there is specific biology that allows
for that sort of relationship. But the fact that there is a specific biology of religiosity does not rule in—or rule out—God," says Boston
University's Patrick McNamara, director of the Evolutionary
Neurobehavior Laboratory.[2]

For the believer, McNamara offers a helpful caution. We must be
careful not to use science as a proof text for our faith. And yet it is astounding that science has discovered this capacity in the human brain.
Through scientific research we are gaining a fuller understanding of

how our bodies work, and this research is telling a fascinating story: our body's design enables us to commune with God and to fellowship more closely with others. As we understand that design, we can even learn to take up the practices that help us to most closely follow God.

No scientific study will ever prove or disprove the existence of God. But the research is quickly accumulating: our bodies, down to our cells and our DNA, are designed for spiritual experience. For those who understand themselves as made in the image of God, this research can be life changing. Not only is God interested in our intellectual or emotional connection to him; he has designed our bodies to intimately participate in this relationship, to connect to him and to the people around us.

I came to write this book about life, oddly enough, by looking at death. I spent several years working in a funeral home and as a hospice volunteer and quickly found that our culture's discomfort with the body often made loved ones' mourning complex and difficult.

After a person's death, for example, many people held minimalist memorials or "celebration" services, using the funeral home simply as a service to deal with the body for cremation or burial. But a service that simply celebrated life without fully acknowledging death and grief often left families lost in a sea of unexpected emotions after the stream of casseroles ended.

In contrast, acknowledging death and working through grief often required dealing with a dead body. There were some people— and some churches who helped these people—who handled this overwhelming job better than others. These families usually chose observances that suggest the body matters. They tended not to have casual memorial services but more formal funerals, where the body of the deceased was present. They paid final respects. They didn't say things like "Oh, this body is just a shell." Instead, as earlier Christians did, they treated the body with honor, as though it were made in the image of God. Some even held on to older practices such as washing and dressing a body after death. It's not that a certain kind of funeral is the only way to do it, but my experience suggested that the best ones—those that would later seem to be most meaningful and helpful—treated a body with reverence. There was something about the physical presence of a body that helped those in mourning.

This experience with families and hospice patients left me with the deep impression that our bodies matter, and that they matter spiritually. I explored the implications of that in my previous book, *The Art of Dying*. Somehow our flesh and bones, what we do with them and how we treat them, make a difference to us in ways that we think of as nonmaterial.

We can never fully understand the mysterious connection between flesh and spirit, but this book seeks to celebrate what we are learning. Our bodies, the Bible says, are the temples of God—the place where God lives.

The Bible describes in precise detail how the ancient Israelites built the tabernacle and later the stone temple. It tells us where the wood came from and the different kinds used to line the walls and the floors. It even tells us that no iron tools were used on the building site, creating a kind of quiet busyness as workers labored. Every detail of the temple bespoke its heavenly resident.

In the same way, we can now appreciate how our own bodies, as God's temple, have been constructed. If God's earthly residence was covered in pure gold, how much more valuable are these living, breathing temples! As science opens up to us the rich intricacy of our physical design, I hope that we are able to see our earthly temples as finely and beautifully designed works of art, crafted especially for worship.

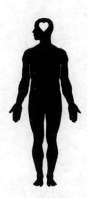

Part One

SPIRITUAL BODIES

PRAYER—THIS IS
YOUR BRAIN ON GOD

EXPECTING PARENTS LOVE NOTHING MORE THAN attending their baby's first ultrasound. There before them, on a simple black-and-white screen, science provides a sneak peek at their long-desired child. The white curve of a backbone with a tiny rib cage. A silhouette of a face marked by mother's nose or father's chin. And a four-chambered heart, beating strong and steady. "It's the only time I'll ever be able to see inside your head," quipped one expectant father to his daughter, warmly cocooned in her mother's womb.

We're fascinated at this intimate look inside another person, the opportunity to see beyond the externals to the inner workings of the body. Because a person is more than just olive skin or blue eyes or slender fingers. It's what's inside that counts.

We can often be tempted to think of our spiritual lives as something external—a collection of things we do: church attendance, Bible reading, prayer, service. Or it is a set of beliefs that we hold. However, our relationship with God is profoundly connected to what is happening inside of us, in our bodies. Experiences of God, ranging from typical feelings of devotion while singing praises to God to the ultimate transcendent union with God, have an impact on the rest of our bodies. These experiences can affect everything from our health to our relationships.

The brain plays a leading role in these spiritual encounters with God. Certainly our relationship with God is much more than a matter of brain waves, but it *includes* brain activity. Here a distinction must be made. The brain is the physical material that scientists can observe. It is the collection of neurons firing back and forth, the chemicals that lubricate those cellular interactions, and the blood flowing to keep it all working. In contrast, the mind is what can't be seen on an MRI or through any other tool of science. The mind is the collection of thoughts and feelings carried by those cells and chemicals. It is our sense of meaning and purpose, our desires and rationalizations. The brain is like the apparatus upon which the mind works.

It must not be thought, however, that the brain and mind are like a computer's hardware and software, as though they could be separated by a computer whiz. On the contrary, the Bible seems to talk about people not as separable parts but as whole beings, with each part affecting other parts. That's what the latest research is showing too. It is as though the hardware of the brain can rewrite the software of the mind. Our behaviors and our actions can change the nature of our brain, which can change the content of our thoughts. At the same time, our very thoughts can cause the neurons in our brain to grow and change.

Through cutting-edge research, as we look inside the brain at work we can catch a sneak peek into God's design of our bodies to commune with him. In doing so we can understand more fully *how* we connect with God and the ways in which we can grow in our spiritual lives.

An Inside Peek

Using the latest brain-imaging technology available, Andrew Newberg, a leading neuroscientist at Thomas Jefferson University Hospital and Medical College in Pennsylvania and professor of religious studies at the University of Pennsylvania, has extensively studied the brain and spiritual experience. The brain, says Newberg, is an intricate system that is "uniquely constructed to perceive and generate spiritual realities."[1]

What would we then see if we could peek in on our brains while praying or meditating on God? The nervous system is a web, running from the brain down through the spinal cord and out to every inch of the body. Its two basic states, "fight or flight" (sympathetic) and "relaxation" (parasympathetic), are responsible for different automatic body processes, like digestion, blood pressure and sweat. Prayer normally tends to enhance the relaxation response, which is why it reduces stress and lowers blood pressure.[2]

However, in intense prayer or in communal worship, both systems can be active at once. "Generally speaking, it is rare that an experience both arouses and calms," says Newberg, "which is one of the reasons why we think spiritual experience stimulates the brain in a unique way."[3] For example, worship can be loud and exciting while also creating a sense of inner peace. Or it may be intellectually stimulating while being relaxing, not taxing. The more that the two systems are simultaneously engaged, the more profound the experience. And when this spiritual circuit is fully engaged, we can experience a feeling of union with God and often with other people as well. In these moments, Newberg says, it is as though "the boundaries between you and God dissolve." And you experience union with God.[4]

In prayer there are other brain systems at work, because spirituality draws on every part of who we are. Our frontal lobe is rationally thinking about the experience, understanding it in terms of theology and application. The limbic system helps to provide an emotional flavor to the experience. At the same time, the amygdala, which is often the center of our experiences of fear and anger, might be soothed or calmed.[5] Our anterior cingulate would help to translate these thoughts and emotions into compassion and empathy toward other people.[6]

These structures of the brain are highly active during a spiritual experience. While the brain is engaged in an unusual way, it also seems to be functioning normally. Some have argued that spirituality is a hallucination or caused by epilepsy. But unlike those dysfunctions, spirituality seems to enhance the brain's capacity in a number of ways, it has healthful effects on the rest of the body, and it is personally meaningful.

Within the structures of the brain run chemicals that play vital roles in spiritual experiences like prayer. The neurons of the brain communicate through neurotransmitters, chemicals that send messages across the synapse (gap) between two cells. Even these chemicals are part of our spiritual experience and play an important role in our body's ability to connect with God. For example, researchers have found that the neurotransmitter serotonin is typically released during intense spiritual experience. Serotonin is produced by nerve cells in the brain as well as in the gut. The amount of serotonin in your brain can elevate your mood as well as affect memory, learning, sleep and vision. A healthy level of serotonin and you're happy as a clam. Low levels of serotonin and your physician might recommend taking an antidepressant medication.

In one study, Dr. Franz Vollenweider, director of the Heffter Research Institute in Zurich, Switzerland, found that blocking serotonin in the brain caused his research subjects to struggle with having spiritual experiences. Individuals remarked that they could not experience God.[7]

Certainly the ability to have a spiritual experience cannot be isolated to a single brain chemical. There is no shortage of Christian saints who suffered depression—and probably low levels of serotonin—and yet were close to God. But research does indicate that neurotransmitters play an important role in how we experience God. And conversely, these studies may help us to better understand times when we feel God's absence. The "dark night of the soul" may be not simply a form of spiritual depression but a signal that the brain is changing. One researcher believes that spiritual experiences can be so powerful that they knock loose some of the brain's wiring, creating a sense of God's absence as the brain rewires the necessary parts to experience God. In these periods of life, we may know cognitively that God exists but find it hard to connect with him. Whether we suffer from chronic depression or have an occasional case of the blues, serotonin levels are diminished, and that can affect our spiritual lives.

More Than a Feeling

If the design of our brain can allow for the lows of doubt or depression, it also provides amazing capacity for powerfully intimate connections with God. Mario Beauregard, a neuroscientist at the University of Montreal, conducted brain scans of Carmelite nuns while they recalled their spiritual experiences and saw this occurring with startling regularity. In one experiment, he studied fifteen nuns during three separate brain states: resting, then while remembering an intense feeling of union with another human being, and finally as they recalled an experience of union with God.

We might expect that remembering these two kinds of emotional experiences would involve similar brain systems. Yet in Beauregard's research, remembering an experience of God proved to be unique. Beauregard found that the mystical state involved areas of the brain that orient the body in space. In remembering intimacy with God, the nuns' brains responded not simply with a feeling of relational connection but with a strong sense of union to something beyond themselves. Several of the women "mentioned that during the Mystical condition they felt the presence of God, His unconditional and infinite love, as well as plenitude and peace."[8] While both kinds of union involved strong feelings, spirituality was a unique experience in the brain.

Intense spiritual experiences cause the brain to work in ways that suggest spirituality is a specific capability of our brains. Beauregard says his studies confirm that spiritual experiences involve far more than the emotional parts of the brain, including "a variety of functions, such as self-consciousness, emotion, body representation, visual and motor imagery, and spiritual perception."[9]

Finally, God has designed our brains with the ability to change, to be transformed. The apostle Paul exhorts believers to "be transformed by the renewing of your mind" (Rom 12:2). This isn't just a nice suggestion. Andrew Newberg and Mark Robert Waldman write, "Intense, long-term contemplation of God . . . appears to permanently change the structure of those parts of the brain that control our moods, give rise to our conscious notions of self, and shape our sensory perceptions of the world."[10] As our brains change—literally with neurons growing, adapting, knitting themselves together—the brain area that deals with anger becomes less active, and compassion for others grows.[11] Our memory is enhanced, we become more motivated, and our baseline level of happiness increases. We become generally more joyful.

This improved neural functioning can help our general health. "Spiritual practices," says Newberg, "enhance the neural functioning of the brain in ways that improve physical and emotional health."[12] As we regularly commune with God, we create the neural pathways that strengthen our relationship, eliminating those things that would detract from our growth and reinforcing and developing those habits that lead to our sanctification. This is how God designed us to thrive.

Practicing Prayer

Prayer can look like lots of different things. It can be chatty, meditative, stream of consciousness, or focused. But researchers tell us that the kind of prayer that changes our brains is a specific kind: deep prayer, or focused, attentive prayer. And many of us are not accustomed to this kind of prayer.

Prayer that changes us involves our full concentration. Fair warning: this sort of prayer often doesn't come easily. Evelyn Underhill, a twentieth-century writer on Christian mysticism, considers how difficult attentive prayer can be. "The first quarter of an hour thus spent in attempted meditation will be, indeed, a time of warfare; which should at least convince you how unruly, how ill-educated is your attention, how miserably ineffective your will, how far away you are from the captaincy of your own soul."[13]

This style of prayer is hard because so much of our life is built on distraction. To hear the "still small voice" of God, we need to quiet our minds. And if prayer is going to change us, we need to pay attention, close attention, to God and our own hearts.

Christian history provides us with many methods for attentive, focused prayer. Many Christians still practice the centuries-old method of the spiritual exercises or daily examen taught by Ignatius of Loyola. Others find the contemplative prayer of the desert fathers and mothers and *lectio divina* from the Benedictines to be helpful methods of prayerful contemplation. Since the 1970s, centering prayer has also provided guidance to Christians looking to focus their hearts through prayer. These guides, and others, all call the Christian to quiet her mind, remove herself from the cares and noise of the day, and simply sit in God's presence.

In contrast, many Protestant methods are heavy on content, encouraging those in prayer to use the skills often used in classrooms or Bible study. While we ought to be filling our minds with biblical teaching, learning to listen to God requires that we be still and, sometimes, stop talking. For example, the ACTS pattern of prayer (adoration, confession, thanksgiving, supplication) can keep our minds too busy, at times preventing us from becoming quiet and attentive. It's a great pattern of prayer but may not be the best model for leading us into the kind of communion with God that we seek.

Pray, Learn, Repeat

If we are to pray in ways that shape our brains, we must be willing to practice. Because of my busy family and work life, it is always a challenge to find a time when I can avoid distraction for a full fifteen minutes. Of late, I have found that space as I sit in the dark in my children's bedroom after I tuck them in at night. While they lie quietly waiting for sleep to come, I set my timer and begin to pray. They like the companionship as they drift off to sleep; I appreciate the opportunity to practice quiet prayer. And when it's hard to calm the restlessness in my mind, the timer allows me to pray for a specific period without checking every few minutes to see how much time I have left.

Sitting with my back against the wall, I begin by quietly saying the name of Jesus. I pray in whispers, because it helps my concentration to be moving my lips and hearing my own prayer. Praying solely in my mind too easily allows me to become distracted.

After a few minutes of saying Jesus' name, I have "warmed up" and entered a prayerful mental posture, one that allows me to be filled with Scripture and truth. I then pray, again by repetition, phrases from the Psalms that I have learned through instruction or ones that I particularly like: "Bless the Lord, O my soul" or "God is my refuge and strength." Sometimes I repeat phrases from written prayers, such as "Come, Lord Jesus, draw me to yourself," and the Jesus Prayer, "Lord Jesus Christ, Son of God, have mercy on me." I often try to picture a biblical scene while I pray. I find this also helps my concentration.

As I sit in the quiet dark, I find I am easily distracted. Even while I am praying, my mind wanders elsewhere, thinking about what happened during the day, things I must do, or concerns I have. That's bound to happen, though, and I simply keep refocusing my attention.

Sometimes the buzz of the timer is a relief—focus has been difficult to find that night. Other times I am surprised that the time has passed so quickly. Once my timer goes off, I begin to pray for specific things. I find that my conversation with God about my hopes, worries and concerns is much livelier and spiritually sensitive after I have spent fifteen minutes in attentive prayer.

Other methods, such as *lectio divina* and praying through written prayers, have allowed me to expand the language of my prayer life. When I use *lectio divina*, I pray slowly and methodically over a short biblical passage. My intent isn't to study and understand the meaning of the text in an exegetical way, but simply to allow the inspired Word of God to speak. Memorizing written prayers such those in the Book of Common Prayer also has allowed me to enter into a deeper and more focused prayer.

Thomas Merton wrote, "I pray better to You by walking than by talking." His words resonate with me as a student of attentive prayer. During regular walks, I can repeat the Jesus Prayer or "Come, Lord Jesus." I enter a rhythm in which my prayer, my breathing and my walking flow together. When I pray on a walk, I find that my mood shifts significantly even though my mind seems to take on a heightened awareness of the trees, the landscaping, or my direction. My attention to my prayer has caused a subconscious adjustment.

Effects likes these extend to my children as well. Praying like this can dismantle a temper tantrum. It can help an energized child settle into bed and fall fast asleep. In our home, attentive prayer has ended sleepwalking sessions, calmed tears and fears, and soothed nightmares. While children may be less able to assert rational control over their moods, prayer offers them a tool to calm and settle the mind and an intimate access to relationship with God.

What I can witness in my children I know is also true of me. Focused, attentive prayer changes me and allows me to experience God in a way that other forms of worship cannot. It changes who I am at a deeper level than I can reach through direct, intentional efforts to try to be more compassionate or to let go of anger or jealousy. It enables me to follow the words of Scripture long after I have left the quiet fifteen minutes in my children's bedroom.

It's Not All in Your Head

When Paul encourages the Ephesians toward Christian living, he includes two powerful categories of change. His admonition to "be made new in the attitude of your minds" is quickly followed by a list of dos and don'ts for social relationships (Eph 4:23). He gives instructions on lying, stealing, gossip, generosity and forgiveness. Paul clearly saw that internal change comes hand in hand with external change. For Paul, and for neuroscientists who study brain activity today, the connection between what we think and what we do is a powerful one.

The brain activity of our spiritual life involves not only private piety but public concern as well. We are designed both to love God and to love our neighbor. From the habits of our minds to prayer to deep relationships and acts of service, we can take steps to become people who are in touch with God.

Researchers have found that spiritual activity, such as prayer, enhances our brain's ability to recognize the suffering of others and to respond in action. The areas of the brain involved in spirituality tend to strengthen those involved in compassion. Prayer, this research shows, helps us control feelings like anger and fear and helps us feel connected to other people. By praying with another person, or even *for* another person while alone, research shows that we can ease negative feelings and enhance our connection to that person.

The anterior cingulate is a backward-C-shaped brain structure that sits a few inches behind the forehead. This region is involved in regulating bodily activities like blood pressure and heart rate, but it is also involved in emotion, the expectation of rewards and empathy. Researchers have found this area of the brain is involved in prayer and meditation as well as compassion. Since neurons are like muscles—the more they work the stronger they are—exercising this area in prayer enhances a person's compassion.

Researchers compared the responses of expert meditators and novices to distressful sounds. When both groups were at rest or meditating, they found that the anterior cingulate and another brain region, the insula, were the most affected by these noises. They also found that the longtime meditators responded more strongly, and those expert meditators who said "they had successfully entered into the meditative state" tended to respond *most* strongly.[14]

Other studies have confirmed and amplified these results, finding that within a relatively short amount of time a person's compassion can grow through meditation. Another study gave subjects thirty minutes of online meditation training for fourteen days. They split the subjects into two groups; one group practiced "compassion meditation" while the other control group engaged in "cognitive training." At the end of the fourteen days, subjects were asked whether they wanted to donate part of the money they received from participating in the study to charitable causes. The compassion meditators, especially those "who showed the biggest boost in activity in the insula," were more compassionate than those who participated in cognitive training. The insula is located near the center of each hemisphere of the brain, and part of its function is to regulate social emotions as well as mind and body interactions.The paticipants with a more active insula donated the most money.[15]

The fact that prayer and compassion are so interrelated in the brain helps us to understand the apostle John's assertion that as we love one another, "[God's] love is made complete in us" (1 Jn 4:11-12).

Neuroscience and the Soul

Our culture tends to reduce all things to matter, and more and more aspects of our lives are being "demystified" of the spiritual qualities they were once assumed to have. What in centuries past was a universe alive with God's Spirit we now see as driven by mechanical forces. If we see our own spiritual nature as the simple result of these biological forces, we become products of the mere mechanics of the universe. Part of our challenge is to get past the only options our culture can envision, either of mechanical nature or of an external, supernatural spiritual force that is able to break the laws of nature. We find this struggle particularly true when we look at science and ask: Where is the soul? Do we have a soul?

The Bible's approach can help us get beyond this dichotomy. It doesn't seem much concerned about whether we are made of two parts (body and soul) or three (body, soul and spirit). Its original audiences and writers were more concerned with what a thing was for (its function), rather than what it was made of (its composition), says John Walton, an Old Testament professor at Wheaton College. He writes, "People in the ancient world [including the original readers and writers of the Old and New Testaments] believed that something existed not by virtue of its material properties, but by virtue of its having a function in an ordered system."[16] As a result, we don't find in the Bible a list of ingredients for a human being, though we read many instructions for how a human being should act.

If we see the Bible's description of humanity through functions, things can become clearer. In the New Testament we see Greek words like *sarx* (body or flesh), *nous* (mind), *pneuma* (spirit), *kardia* (heart) and *psyche* (soul). These are not so much building blocks of who we are as things we do. We are people who will die and return to dust, so we are corruptible flesh waiting to put on incorruption (in Paul's words in 1 Cor 15:53). We are also animated by the breath of God (spirit); we think rationally (mind) and feel (heart), and we have a personhood (soul). These aren't puzzle pieces that can be pulled apart and fit back together. Instead, says N. T. Wright, "When Paul thinks of human beings he sees every angle of vision as contributing to the whole, and the whole from every angle of vision. All lead to the one, the one is seen in the all."[17] It would seem that our composition is more like a long-simmering jambalaya, where the flavors of the ingredients blend together, than a ham sandwich with the cheese slipping out from between the ham and bread.

This Is Your Brain on God

In 1987, the US antinarcotics group Partnership for a Drug Free America introduced what would become one of the most memorable commercials in television. Audiences saw an egg drop into a hot frying pan, heard the sizzle, and were told, "This is your brain on drugs. Any questions?"

The spot was memorable not only because it was an emotionally compelling piece but also because it confirmed a popular view that drugs can fry your brain. Nicole Dudukovic, a memory researcher in human biology at Stanford, recalls, "I didn't really understand how my brain would ever be anything remotely like a fried egg, but I certainly got the message that drugs weren't good for me."[18]

New research arrives yearly in scientific journals expanding and clarifying our understanding of this most fascinating organ. Explaining brain functioning is certainly a complex endeavor; exploring the interaction between our bodies and an unseen God is even more so.

The three parts of this book are designed to reveal more about these mysterious, wonderfully made bodies we inhabit. First, we will see how our bodies are spiritual, such as how eating or exercise or hospitality affects us. We will see how from birth we are primed to look for God and connect significantly with the people around us. We will also see how our bodies respond to the people around us throughout our lives, from casual observation to the intimacy of marriage. And we will consider what it means when our bodies malfunction. How do we think of God as Creator when the creation is broken?

Part two will explore how we change through spiritual practices. The spiritual disciplines are sometimes seen as a kind of magic: do this to make that happen. Actually, there are biological reasons that spiritual practices change who we are. Finally, in part three we will see how this all adds up to a fully engaged life, one that is physically healthy and personally meaningful. Because we are not simply individuals on a spiritual journey, we will also consider what Christians living in tune with God and loving their neighbors can offer in a world in which these deepest human needs are so often unmet.

To be sure, this endeavor is a complex one. Perhaps that's why we find metaphors helpful. If your brain on drugs is like an egg in a frying pan, your brain on God is like a harpist playing a beautiful song. In physics, the most fundamental property in the universe is a one-dimensional vibrating string. As we engage in disciplines such as prayer, we tune our hearts to resonate with the Creator. Then just as a vibrating string causes other strings with the same frequency to also vibrate, neuron by neuron begins to respond, working in harmony to create new pathways, so that our brains resound in praise. And these sweet tones cannot help but resonate out to those around us. They ripple out in acts of love and service, the practical workings out of a faith that has begun in the infinitesimally small places of the brain.

BORN CONNECTORS

As a child, I first experienced God at the dinner table. My family gathered nightly around the small round table in our kitchen, and each dinner began with prayer. Often our prayers would circle the table, as each person was given opportunity to pray or praise. On this particular night, I joined in. I cannot remember what we were having for dinner that night. I cannot remember what I prayed. But as we finished and began to pick up our forks, I felt the love of God. It must have been a prayer I felt very seriously about, because I began to cry. My sister asked why I was crying, but my mother wisely knew I'd experienced the Lord. She reached over and rubbed my back, reassuring me that tears were an okay response to touching the holy.

We often think of passing our faith on to our children as something we do by educating them in Bible stories and instructing them in values and morals in preparation for the time when they will make a personal commitment to Jesus. Yet we may not realize that the most important aspect of nurturing children in the faith is to offer them the chance to directly experience God and the love of God through the community of his people. Research is now showing that children are born equipped with a predisposition for a belief in God and a capacity for spiritual experiences. Spirituality is inborn and ready for action from surprisingly early ages.

Today researchers have learned that children are not blank slates upon which parents and other adults can write any kind of instruction. Babies are born with certain expectations about and needs from the world around them. As they grow, children need formative connections with other people, and they expect to discover God.

Primed for Belief

Justin Barrett is the director of the Thrive Center for Human Development at Fuller Seminary and a former researcher at Oxford's Centre for Anthropology and Mind. He focuses his research on children's spirituality, and through his research and that of others Barrett has discovered that children are primed to believe in God and spiritual beings. In fact, these beliefs appear to be hardwired into children when they are born. While these beliefs and inclinations cannot be isolated to a particular gene strand or brain chemical, the near-universality of their occurrence leads social scientists to believe that this capacity is the baseline or natural state of all humans.

First, Barrett says that young children know the difference between make-believe fairy tales and reality, and they firmly place spiritual beings, including God, within the realm of the latter. While they might be afraid of monsters under the bed at night, children can distinguish in the light of day that these things do not exist. In contrast, they believe in the reality of Jesus even though he is not visible to their eyes.

Second, children attribute intention and purpose to the world they see. Ask a child why a mountain exists, and the child will give his own reason for it, even if the scientific process of continental shift has been explained to him. Children will say that the mountains are there to look pretty, so that the bears can climb on them, or so that people can go skiing. They are not simply interested in the *how* but in the *why* as well. "With these abilities in place in infancy and with a heightened tendency to detect agents or attribute agency in the face of little encouragement, very young children are receptive to the idea of gods; it may even be that were children not provided with ideas about gods, they would discover gods for themselves."[1]

Research by Barrett and others suggests that children are even rather sophisticated in their theological concepts. As early as age four, children know that their parents have not created the world around them, even though children attribute superhuman abilities to their parents. Likewise, children have expectations about the world from which they cannot be easily dissuaded. In other words, religious parents are not able to simply inculcate any set of religious beliefs in their children. We "underestimate how much information children are born already having or are predisposed to acquire easily and rapidly," Barrett says. Children learn religious ideas more easily because they have hardwired expectations about spiritual influences in the world. Barrett even argues that it can be difficult to "indoctrinate children away from religious belief."[2]

These studies seem to indicate that our children may be more able to comprehend spiritual things than we have previously given them credit for. Their brains are hardwired for spiritual experiences, and they have the capacity—however rudimentary—for discerning spiritual realities.

One of the most significant applications of these realities appears in the writings of Sofia Cavaletti, founder of the Catechesis of the Good Shepherd and author of numerous books on children and spiritual formation. In her landmark book *The Religious Potential of the Child,* Cavalletti tells this story:

It is a fact that the child seems capable of seeing the Invisible, almost as if it were more tangible and real than the immediate reality. Bianca (five and a half years old) was mixing flour with yeast, as an exercise relating to the parable that compares the Kingdom of God to the yeast that leavens the dough. The catechist asked her to explain to a woman who had come to visit the center what she was doing; Bianca responded: "I am watching how the Kingdom of God grows." . . . Children penetrate effortlessly beyond the veil of signs and "see" with utmost facility their transcendent meaning, as if there were no barrier between the visible and the Invisible.[3]

Scottie May is a professor of Christian formation at Wheaton College and for decades has studied the spiritual lives of children. She has seen this research play out in Sunday school classrooms and children's worship experiences. In an interview she told me, "Children are spiritual and are able to fall in love with Jesus at age two or three or four." May found that they were able to grasp theological concepts concerning God and eternity, rudimentary in form, perhaps, but with an understanding perfectly appropriate for their age.

After years of working with children, researching their spiritual capacities and talking with adults about their formative spiritual experiences, May says, "They can have a real relationship with the living God. . . . My goal in working with children is to help them love the Lord Jesus because Jesus loves them so much."

Ready for Connection

Children's neural development primes them for deep connections with God and their neighbors. These deep connections grow rapidly in the first years of life, making deep imprints on the brain and patterns that can last into adulthood.

Our connection to other people begins at birth. At the end of pregnancy, mothers' oxytocin receptors spike in their brains. This chemical is a "feel-good" chemical of the brain, and it assists in social bonding: the female brain is preparing itself to experience extra joy and love as the mother bonds with her new baby.

At the same time, babies are ready to connect to their mothers. Studies have found that when shown pictures of faces, infants just ten minutes old will look at them longer than at similar patterns that are not faces. "A newborn's brain *expects* faces," says neuroscientist David Eagleman.[4] Researcher Paul Zak explains in *The Moral Molecule* that these expectations grow into mimicry as children receive and send out social cues. "Open your mouth and they'll open their mouth. Stick out your tongue and they'll do the same. They're trying on these social gestures, working to master them and weave them into their neural wiring."[5]

These brain developments aren't just psychological in value, however. They also have measurable physical benefits. One study showed that when premature babies were regularly massaged, they gained 47 percent more weight than their nursery neighbors who did not get massages. Other than the massage, their care and nutrition were the same. But the massaged babies experienced through gentle touch the love and care of others.[6]

The effect goes both ways. When doctors encouraged new mothers to hold their infants, skin to skin, for an hour soon after birth and then for five more hours over the next three days, they found that those mothers were vastly more attuned to their babies. The results even five years later are astonishing. A total of just six hours of skin-to-skin contact in the first three days resulted in mothers who spent more time soothing their babies, caressing them and making eye contact a full month later. One year later, those mothers were found to ask the doctor more questions during an annual checkup. They also helped the doctor more. Two years later, they needed to give their children fewer commands than mothers who hadn't spent that extra time cuddling their babies. Perhaps most shocking is that five years after those six hours of physical contact, those children scored higher on IQ and language tests.[7]

What begins at birth extends into childhood. Children depend on this connection to parents as they head out into the world. When researchers placed one-year-old babies on the edge of a clear glass surface that appeared to be a cliff, 80 percent of the babies would, when encouraged by their mothers, crawl out across what could have been nothing. Every infant checked with Mommy for how to respond to being placed on the edge of the cliff, and more than three-quarters would launch out into apparent nothingness if encouraged to do so. Yet if the mother appeared to be afraid, none of the babies would dare cross it.[8]

In another experiment, scientists told mothers to stop smiling at their children while they played. How did the children respond? They stopped exploring their play area. They ignored new toys and play structures. "The child quickly becomes agitated and distressed, often wildly so, arching his or her back and crying out." The child would try to provoke the mother with both tears and smiles. Failing that, it "falls into listlessness and torpor."[9]

Unfortunately, studies showing us the dark side of this brain development, what happens when a child's brain does not receive this important care, are many. Children who are not nurtured by loving, caring adults grow up to have—among other disadvantages—lower

IQ, lower emotional capacities and worse physical health.

In the late 1950s and 60s, researcher Harry Harlow performed what are now famous experiments on a group of monkeys, depriving them of their natural mother and giving them a wire mesh "mother" and another wire mother covered in terrycloth. Depending on the experiment, Harlow dispensed food through a bottle provided by one or both of the mothers. He found that the baby monkeys preferred the terrycloth mother, whether or not they provided food, suggesting touch is a more fundamental need than nutrition. He then took his experiment further, depriving some infant monkeys of social contact. One group was able to see, hear and smell other monkeys but never make social contact. Another group was completely isolated.[10]

Harlow's discoveries overturned the prevailing idea of the time that children needed nourishment but not touch. By showing the horrible effects of social isolation, Harlow helped put to rest the behavioral theories that dominated psychology—though behaviorist ideas still reign in popular thought today. Monkeys who were deprived only of touch tended to self-mutilate, they repeatedly circled their cages, and they stared blankly into space. But the socially isolated monkeys were in far worse shape. They were never able to reintegrate into a social group. Introducing them to others caused total shock. Many died. Others would hold and cradle themselves, rocking constantly.

Thankfully, Harlow's experiments were never performed on human babies. However, some orphanages have offered a horrifying "natural experiment." The Bucharest Early Intervention Project researched the effects of institutionalization and neglect in orphanages in Romania in the 1990s after the fall of dictator Nicolae Ceausescu and found profound delays in children who were deprived of nurturing care in their early years of life.[11] The world was shocked to see pictures of children who had spent their childhood years literally caged in these institutions. We now know that depriving infants of love and physical affection can cause permanent damage to the brain. Because of those tragedies, we can now see what exactly goes wrong in the brain when neglect impairs development.

A range of studies have found that institutionalized children tend to develop less white and less gray matter in the brain. White matter is the supportive cell structures that allow the brain's neurons to do their processing. One experiment found that the white matter did not develop properly around areas of the brain that have to do with logical thinking, memory formation and emotional processing. Apparently certain chemicals needed to produce those cells are missing when children are left in isolation. Research on mice has found that there is a certain period during which this white matter must develop; otherwise it never will.[12] The Romanian orphans also had less gray matter—thinking neurons—in their brains. Without vital human interaction, the developing brain fails to work properly, and that failure can be permanently damaging, making future social interaction complex and difficult.

Spiritual Influences Retained

Children are born with an innate sensitivity toward spiritual things and a longing for deep connectedness to others around them, but faith is not born merely of predispositions but of active commitment. The conundrum of "good Christian kids" who leave their faith when they enter adulthood has produced an outpouring of studies examining the faith of teens and young adults to determine what makes faith work. Why do some children filled with knowledge of God and embraced by caring nurture turn their backs on the faith of their parents? Why does one child's faith experience become impossible to reject while another's becomes impossible to accept?

Scottie May and coauthor Catherine Stonehouse paint a picture of a childhood experience of God that may form the soul into adulthood. For Stonehouse and May, a child's brain and social developments blossom best when they are surrounded by a familylike community where multiple generations offer models of a lived-out faith and where all the adults take an interest in children's spiritual growth. This nurturing community offers a path toward knowing God, not just learning about God. "On the way of *experience* children are most likely to meet God and come to know God deeply."[13] Statistically speaking, according to Barna, children who maintained their faith into adulthood were twice as likely to have had a close relationship with an adult at church. Nearly 60 percent of church kids who kept their faith into adulthood had such a friendship.[14]

In their book *Sticky Faith*, Kara Powell and Chap Clark report on their extensive study on what makes faith last. They find three traits of the kind of faith nurtured by adults. "Sticky faith" is internal and external; that is, it involves behaviors like church attendance and Bible reading that are combined with inner emotional commitment. It is personal and communal; that is, such faith involves an individual relationship with God, but it is anchored in a supportive community. Finally, sticky faith is "mature and maturing"; that is, it "shows the marks of spiritual maturity but is also in the process of growth."[15] For these little ones with rapidly developing brains, a nurturing community carries them along, providing a safe place for their spiritual lives to grow at a natural pace with their physical, emotional and mental development.

Un-Christian? Take Hope

Generation Ex-Christian, Almost Christian, unChristian, Soul Searching, Sticky Faith: the books written to report on, explain and offer antidotes to the number of Christian young people who are leaving the faith are now sagging the bookshelves of youth pastors around the country. As a parent, I'm also anxious that my children grow up to become responsible adults and stick with their faith in Jesus, even as they must develop their own relationship with God and understanding of what it means to be a Christian.

A lot of young people who grew up in the church struggle to sustain that faith once they are out on their own. According to the Barna Group, as many as six in ten young adults who had been active in youth group as teenagers disengage from church to a significant degree and often for a long time.[16] And probably under half of those kids who leave the church end up returning (estimates range from 30 to 60 percent).[17] It used to be that marriage and children would send those who had left the faith back, but now that people spend so many of their adult years single and unattached, finding their way back to faith after fifteen years away isn't so easy.

It can often feel that our culture's obstacles to a faithful Christian life are immense: materialism, violent and sexualized entertainment, relegation of faith to a strictly private and personal sphere, and hostility to faith from certain cultural quarters. All these and more can make it seem an incredibly difficult task to nurture a child into adulthood with a faith that remains strong.

But the research I've been examining in this chapter should give us hope. If inclinations toward faith are in some degree hardwired, then parents have some advantages. It isn't easy to stamp out faith.

Throughout Scripture, God speaks to children and teens. Mary is believed to have been just a girl, thirteen or fourteen years old,

when the angel visited her and announced that she would give birth
to a boy. The spirituality of children is taken for granted in Scripture.
"The boy Samuel ministered before the LORD," begins 1 Samuel 3.
Scholars believe he would have been about twelve years old when
God first called him by name and Samuel mistook God's voice for
that of Eli the priest. The chapter concludes, "The LORD was with
Samuel as he grew up, and he let none of Samuel's words fall to the
ground. And all Israel from Dan to Beersheba recognized that
Samuel was attested as a prophet of the LORD. The LORD continued
to appear at Shiloh, and there he revealed himself to Samuel
through his word" (1 Sam 3:19-21).

In cultures where Christian faith has been nearly extinguished,
spiritual beliefs have remained. In Europe, a continent where only
52 percent of citizens say they believe in God, Estonia is one of the
least religious societies. Eighteen percent of Estonians say they believe in God.[18] The largest religious group is Lutheran, and only 13
percent of the population says they practice the faith.[19] Yet only a
quarter of Estonians are strictly atheist and say there is no God.
Fifty-four percent of the population believes in some kind of spiritual force, and self-described pagan nature worship is common.[20]

Sociologists Rodney Stark and Roger Finke say what has died in
Europe is not faith but a state church. "Levels of subjective reli-
giousness remain high," they write. "To classify a nation as highly
secularized when the large majority of its inhabitants believe in
God is absurd. Indeed, the important question about religion in
Europe is . . . not why people no longer believe, but why they 'persist
in believing but see no need to participate with even minimal regularity in their religious institutions.'" Stark and Finke write that
there is actually very little difference between Europeans and
Americans when researchers look at people's beliefs on each con-

tinent. In Iceland, for example, where just 2 percent of the population goes to church, more than 80 percent believe in a soul and pray at least sometimes outside of church.[21]

In the United States, where a rapidly growing percent of the population claims no affiliation to traditional religion, roughly 68 percent of these nonreligious say they are pretty sure there is a God. And 40 percent pray at least monthly. These "religiously unaffiliated" are religious in a variety of ways. They pray and seek out spiritual activities, but—like Europeans—they don't consider themselves to be a part of a particular religious group.[22]

However official religious observance changes, people continue to believe in God or gods, and they engage in spiritual practices. They are hardwired to do so. As neuroscientist Andrew Newberg says, "The fact remains that every human brain, from early childhood on, contemplates the possibility that spiritual realms exist."[23]

The question is then how to make specifically Christian faith attractive as children become adults. One primary way, as we have seen, is for young Christians to have meaningful relationships with older ones. We are born connectors, and our spirituality also has a communal aspect. Intergenerational relationships—and acts of service—provide strong ties to the faith of one's youth. Perhaps these relationships allow young Christians to express their doubts and concerns more freely than with parents and pastors. Perhaps they have the opportunity to see how adults outside of their own family connect their beliefs to their lives. Young Christians may simply be better able to see active faith in adults who are not their parents.

Whatever the reason, parents and church leaders can be confident knowing that even though today there may be more challenges and obstacles to maintaining one's childhood faith as an adult, we are wired for faith.

Nurtured from the Cradle

In 1735 John Wesley boarded a ship bound for Georgia with a group of Moravian Brethren. When a storm began to churn on the Atlantic, Wesley watched in awe as his shipmates calmly sang and prayed. Wesley wrote, "The sea broke over, split the main-sail in pieces, covered the ship, and poured in between the decks, as if the great deep had already swallowed us up. A terrible screaming began among the English. The Germans [Moravians] calmly sung on. I asked one of them afterwards, 'Was you not afraid?' He answered, 'I thank God, no.'" After that experience, Wesley sought out the kind of inner confidence he saw in the Moravians and later found it one night when his heart was "strangely warmed" by the reality of the gospel.

However, Wesley was no Jonah fleeing from God's calling for his life. He was sailing to America to be a missionary! This warming of his heart wasn't an adult conversion but the maturing of fruit planted in his childhood. John Wesley's faith had been nurtured from the cradle.

Wesley's father was absent for much of his life, and his mother—a strong, stubborn and brilliant woman—thought that her ten children were not receiving an adequate upbringing in the faith from their local rector. So Susanna Wesley began her own Sunday afternoon services for her family. They quickly attracted as many as two hundred neighbors. Susanna's husband was embarrassed because he too was a rector in the parish, despite spending most of his time in London. It put him in an odd spot to have his wife officiate services at his house because those at his church were deemed inadequate for his own family.

In a letter to her appalled husband, Susanna defended her right to nurture their children's spiritual lives. She wrote, "As to it looking particular, I grant it does. And so does everything that is serious or that may any way advance the glory of God or the salvation of souls if it be performed out of a pulpit, or in the way of common conversation, because in our corrupt age, the utmost care and diligence have to be used to banish all discourse of God or spiritual concerns out of our society."[24]

John Wesley is known to have controversially preached outside of the setting of the church. "The world is my parish," he said. Yet he only did what he had seen his mother, Susanna, doing. John Wesley's disciplined faith in pursuit of holiness was not his own discovery. His lively faith and life of service had strong roots in the nurture of his mother in his childhood years. Surely in his childhood Wesley had listened closely at his mother's knee. His body had been designed in the womb to connect with God, and his mother's wise nurture laid down vital neural pathways that would prepare him to respond to the prompting of the Holy Spirit.

MONKEY SEE,
MONKEY DO

MY FRIEND CHRIS IS A QUALITY manufacturing expert with a
track record of improving the efficiency of large businesses. He has
operated factories, call centers and company-wide quality assurance programs for large publicly traded businesses and has
served as the chief operating officer for a large family-owned
business. Chris loves "lean" businesses; he has a keen eye for taking
the most complex business system and making it simpler, better
and more efficient. He can aggressively cut costs and pinpoint
wasteful spending inside every spreadsheet, all with an eye toward
pursuing higher quality.

You might think that all this focus on process standardization
and quality would mean attention to flow charts and spreadsheets,
an analytical outlook. But Chris believes a more pastoral approach
results in success. For Chris, quality *relationships* form the integral
foundation for a quality product. After all, the perfect flowchart
means nothing if two managers are at odds with each other. Chris
works hard to make sure his employees have responsibilities that
help them to thrive. He wants different departments working together smoothly, and he works hard to end the kinds of turf battles

that can emerge in any organization. He seeks to understand the motives behind what people say in a meeting, not simply to discern whether their ideas are good ones.

On the way home from work each day, I get to see Chris's relational acumen in action as we debrief on the day's events in our carpool. In particular, I've found, he has a knack for reading the emotional content of situations. One day, as a number of us were heading to the elevators, people were cracking jokes about their work. They poked fun at their own weaknesses, and they joked about who would eventually have to fix a problem in their department. As we walked down the hallway, rode the elevator and headed out into the parking lot, a constant rumble of laughs accompanied us, along with discussions about work and questions about family and weekend plans.

"Did you feel that?" Chris asked me as we got into the car. "*That's* what I'm trying to do here." Chris saw it as a significant goal to cultivate healthy, trusting, enjoyable relationships among people who experienced the joy of work.

Another time Chris stopped by my cube after a long meeting in which very little was achieved. He was a little frustrated that he hadn't been able to work through his agenda, but he also understood that something more important needed his attention. "Linda needed to feel valued," he said. He sensed that her presentation suggested that she was trying to prove her value to the organization, so he had spent most of the meeting showing appreciation for her work. Having recognized her insecurity, he sought to affirm that she filled a valuable place in the organization.

"Did you feel that?" Neuroscientists are showing that we pick up on a person's emotional state by feeling it ourselves, exactly what Chris was doing as he sat in the board room or stood in the elevator with colleagues. Because we feel before we consciously think—in fact our feelings drive our thinking—Chris was more insightful than he understood. The process works something like this. Specific neurons in our brains mimic, or mirror, what we see another person doing. This mimicry provides the basis for our conscious interpretation—our thoughts—about what we are seeing or hearing. Like a person who watches herself waving in a mirror, we are able to decode the words and actions of others only as we reflect them. These kinds of feelings are a fundamental source of our conscious thought. We feel before we think, and our neurons "feel" by mimicking the people around us.

Mirror Neurons

The English writer Oscar Wilde, author of *The Importance of Being Earnest* and other plays, is believed to have said, "By age forty, everyone has the face he deserves." A sour disposition, in other words, produces a sour-looking face; a generous attitude gives a person a cheerful-looking face. It takes time, but what's on the inside shows on the outside. Today science is giving Wilde some evidence for his claim.

Neurologists have discovered the process by which our brains recognize a person's body language and facial expressions. Before this discovery, it was widely assumed that we understand another person by consciously analyzing what they say through their words and their body language. But it's now clear that isn't how it works. We don't think, *She's smiling; she must be happy.* Instead our brains mirror another person's expressions. It is as we mentally imitate the muscle movements of others that we sense their emotions. It is when our neurons imitate a scowl that we sense someone's disapproval.

In the 1980s, a team of researchers was studying the motor neurons of monkeys in a laboratory. Motor neurons are the first involved in a brain's instructions to move a part of the body. At the time, neuroscientists largely believed that specific areas of the brain were involved in particular tasks, without overlap. The team had implanted electrodes to measure how specific neurons fired when performing certain tasks. By mapping out the motor structure of the brain, the team would better understand the process of turning the thought of an action into actual movement. When a neuron fired, the system would crackle like static on the radio.

One day, between experiments, one of the researchers picked up something in sight of a lab monkey. While the monkey was doing nothing, the speakers let out a crackle. It was as though a beaker had gone flying across the room without anyone throwing it. This wasn't supposed to happen.

For the first time, in that lab, scientists noticed what are today called mirror neurons. These unique cells fire both when one is performing an action (picking up a cup) and when one is observing the action (watching a lab researcher pick up a cup). Further research confirmed what the initial fluke uncovered: some of our motor neurons mirror another's actions, as well as prompt us to perform our own actions.

Pushing the experiment further, the team wondered, could mirror neurons distinguish between different purposes for picking up an object? Could they tell the difference between picking up an apple to eat and picking it up to peel? The researchers trained their monkeys to pick up a piece of food and eat it as well as to pick up a piece of food and place it in a container near the mouth. In the experiment, everything about the two actions—the place of the food, the movement of the monkey's hand—was the same except for where the food ended up. Then the researchers recorded the neuron activity of an observing monkey.[1]

The researchers found that when a monkey watched the two actions, there was an overlap of just 25 percent in neuron activity. About three-quarters of the neurons fired for one action but not the other. This meant that the monkey's mirror neurons recorded not just action but *intent*. The brain was picking up thoughts and motives, not just observable behaviors. Since a monkey's brain works like a human's, it was only a matter of time before mirror neurons were confirmed to exist and work in the same way in human brains.

Mirror neuron researcher Marco Iacoboni writes, "Mirror neurons let us understand the intentions of other people. . . . We understand the mental states of others by simulating them in our brain. . . . Our brains are capable of mirroring the deepest aspects of the minds of others, even at the fine-grained level of a single cell."[2] This discovery was no small thing; science had begun to approach an understanding of human empathy, sympathy and connection.

This was a far cry from the previous scientific understanding of how humans perceive others. The older theory assumed that we used a rational, sometimes conscious and sometimes subconscious, process by which we read and analyzed another person's body language. Certain emotions were encoded in particular gestures or looks. We could know someone was angry when his eyebrows narrowed and the lips tightened. When a friend's eyes widened, eyebrows rose and mouth opened, we could know she was surprised.

As we have now discovered, people understand others by subconsciously imitating them, mimicking them at a minute level of brain activity. One of the most important ways in which babies discover the world around them is by imitating the people they see. Mommy smiles; baby smiles. Mommy coos and so does baby. Daddy laughs and so does baby. Mirror neuron researcher Iacoboni believes that mirror neurons are formed and developed through imitation of others, largely during a baby's development. Through this process of nonstop mimicry, babies learn to differentiate themselves from their parents. It seems paradoxical: we learn to understand ourselves as *different* from others by *imitating* those who are closest to us. In fact, when Iacoboni and his team electronically shut down subjects' mirror neurons, they were able to recognize pictures of friends but not of themselves.

This is a small piece of evidence, but it aligns with the view that we gain self-awareness through those we interact with. "The development of a sense of self is facilitated by rich social contexts," says Iacoboni. He believes our idea of who we are does not flow out of a "true self" deep within. Rather, our self has two components, the self and the other. Who we are is a complex mix of our own nature interacting with—and mimicking—the people around us. But there is no such thing as a complete person in isolation from others. We are a product of who we are with.

The imitation provided by mirror neurons shows us that we can know what another person is thinking or feeling by feeling the same ourselves. We feel the tension in a conversation by tightening our own muscles, clenching our fists. Then the feeling of those flexed muscles, that body state, is relayed back to the brain, and we feel tense.

In a fascinating experiment, researchers asked two groups of people to identify the emotions of people shown in a series of pictures. The key was that members of one group were each holding a pencil between their teeth. Because the pencil prevented that group from mimicking the expressions of the faces pictured, they were far less able to identify the emotions the pictures portrayed. Mimicry precedes recognition, as one researcher described the results of the experiment.[3]

It would seem, then, that the better we are at mimicking others, the better our relationships. Another study found that when an actor intentionally imitated a research subject while playing a game, the subjects reported liking the actor much more than actors who didn't mimic their behavior.[4]

Studies have shown links between the motor areas of the brain where the mirror neurons are located and the emotional processing centers in the limbic system. The research is clear that mirror neurons provide a basis for empathy and compassion toward other people. It is by feeling another person's pain that we understand and respond to her or his needs. It is by experiencing their joy that we celebrate with others.

We do have the faces we deserve, because we are mimicking the emotions of those around us and we are constantly expressing our own to communicate with others. We communicate our internal emotional state not only by the tone of our voice or the words we say but by the movement of the muscles in our faces.

Researchers know that after about twenty-five years of marriage, couples tend to look more alike. Now we know why. A quarter-century of mimicry in order to understand and empathize with each other has a permanent effect on the facial muscles. And the change is greater among couples who report higher marital satis-faction.[5] Our faces echo our thoughts and our reflections of those around us.

Embodied Cognition

While we don't consciously register every facial expression, our brains do recognize and feel them. When our mirror neurons are firing in response to another person's intention, we have a much deeper knowledge of the state of his or her mind. Jacoboni writes, "One of the primary goals of imitation may actually be the facilitation of an embodied 'intimacy' between the self and others during social relations."[6]

We often think of our brain as the computer that operates a robot. Our consciousness is the interface that allows us to access the programming to tell our bodies what to do. But this analogy is terribly wrong. We think with our feelings, and our feelings are nothing more than the state of our bodies. That's why they're called *feel*ings. This is what scientists call embodied cognition. Anger is not an idea but tensed and poised muscles, quickened heartbeat, and respiration. Joy is not the content of our thoughts but the bodily experience we call joyfulness—a peaceful relaxation of our muscles, a smile, a posture of openness. Our bodies do more than feel emotions. As neuroscientist Antonio Damasio has showed, bodily actions precede and guide our cognitive thinking, which overlays the many and more powerful feelings and processes that happen underneath.

Marketing gurus bank on our shopping with our emotions and not our pocketbooks. In response we may try to rationally separate our *felt* needs from our *actual* ones, our emotional responses from our rational ones. But Damasio's research shows that how we feel and how we think are not so easily separated. Many of his patients have lost their emotional capacity because of damage to a particular spot in the brain. But the loss of their emotions didn't make these patients more rational. Instead it made them so hyperrational that they could never come to a conclusion. Damasio's attempt to schedule an appointment with one of these patients provides a perfect illustration of why we need to feel, not just think.

> For the better part of a half hour, the patient enumerated reasons for and against each of the two dates: previous engagements, proximity to other engagements, possible meteorological conditions, virtually anything that one could reasonably think about concerning a simple date. . . . He was now walking us through a tiresome cost-benefit analysis, an endless outlining and fruitless comparison of options and possible consequences.[7]

As it turns out, we need to have a feel for things, a sense of what is right. Our rational minds confirm, adjust and occasionally overrule the prodding of our emotional state. But they depend upon the sense of things that the rest of the brain and the body provide. We feel before we think, and if we don't feel we can't actually think.

If we are to change this embodied cognition, we must take a forceful approach. It's only when we think about and plan to exert intentional, long-term attention toward something that it makes a difference to the rest of our body. For example, trendy diets applied for a few weeks or months rarely result in long-term health and weight loss. Even the contestants on weight-loss reality TV shows rarely keep off all of the weight they shed. As long as they were in an environment where their surroundings made healthy choices easy or even inevitable, their conscious mind didn't have to work too hard; once they leave that environment, healthy choices are much more difficult. The success of a diet relies on constant, steady, long-term attention to changing your behavior, and it's hard, conscious work.

A former pastor of mine often said, "What the heart wants, the will chooses and the mind rationalizes." Pastors, philosophers and those who pay attention to how we behave have long known this to be true. Neuroscientists are simply showing how it works. All of our deep logic, well-thought theology and worldview tend to arise from our desires and our loves rather than shaping them. Our job, then, is to train our desires to love the right things. In the language of neuroscience, we need to get the "reward circuitry" of our brains to fire to images of "love, joy, peace, forbearance, kindness, goodness" (Gal 5:22).

It's Not Like I Can Read Minds

Some people have a unique sensitivity to the needs of their neighbors. Marlena Graves has often had a hunch about a friend or acquaintance that seems almost prophetic to her. Her husband Shawn, a philosophy professor with an analytical bent, has learned to trust Marlena's assessments though he often can't tell how his wife can sense what is going on behind the scenes in another person's life.

Marlena is a social worker and a writer in a small town in Ohio. Less than a year before I interviewed her, she had noticed a couple talking at church. They were a model church family. He was successful professionally and was the chair of the deacon committee, charged with handling the church's care for those in need. "I didn't know them really well," Marlena says. But watching the couple talk during church one day, she said to her husband, "Shawn, I'm telling you, I think that there is something going on there. I can't pinpoint it, but their marriage is not good."

Within a year, the deacon had left his wife for his secretary. Because of the threat of the church's disciplining him, he resigned his membership.

"It's not like I can read minds," Marlena says. "Maybe some of it is intuition, but I can read the state of people's souls." Marlena acknowledges she's not clairvoyant and her hunches aren't always right, but she often realizes that a friend or coworker has more going on in her life than she may be letting on.

Marlena believes that she has an unusual ability to read people's facial expressions. She doesn't see her knack as a kind of ESP but instead as a gift of spiritual discernment. Recognizing that her perception is unusually deep and accurate, Marlena asked God why she had such a gift, which can sometimes be a burden. She understood God's response: "So you can pray for them." Marlena took that as a directive, saying, "This allows Shawn and me to show compassion and pray for people."

While it isn't always enjoyable to feel the hidden needs of other people, Marlena's sensitivity has been a gift in her marriage. She met Shawn as a college student and was quickly attracted to his quiet demeanor and powerful intellect. Marlena describes Shawn as like a *Pride and Prejudice* Mr. Darcy, a quiet and therefore sometimes misunderstood character. His discreet manner may come across as standoffish, but, Marlena says, behind the scenes Shawn actively cares for people in need. As they got to know each other, Marlena says, when she learned she and Shawn shared a love for 1970s Christian musician Keith Green, she was sold. They married shortly after college.

Together they've learned to overcome their different styles of communicating with a special focus on attentiveness. Shawn, the philosopher, is a linear and analytic thinker, while Marlena is a feeler. Shawn narrates the details of an event, moving from point to point to conclusion. Marlena expresses the emotions of an event, how people felt about it and the impressions she gained, leaving the details fuzzy. To connect more deeply with her spouse, Marlena has learned to take more time to process her thoughts and narrate in a more systematic way. Shawn has learned to be satisfied with being told about the feeling of an event, to offer less processed descriptions of events and to let Marlena know how things make him feel.

Because of this conscious, long-term practice in tuning their minds to each other, Shawn and Marlena have grown better able to communicate. They may seem to be wired differently, but by aligning their conscious thoughts and actions with the work already happening in their mirror neurons, Marlena and Shawn are building strong neural patterns that support their life together.

By paying attention and consciously imitating others, we can improve our ability to recognize how others feel and learn to empathize with them. Worried you'll look odd or be seen as a copycat? Studies show that when two strangers interact, they like each other more when mimicking one another's behaviors.

You Already Love Your Neighbor as Yourself

In his Sermon on the Mount, Jesus articulated a fulfillment of God's law that astounded his listeners. "You have heard that it was said," Jesus begins as he explodes the Pharisaic limitations that had been applied to the Ten Commandments: If you curse your brother, it is as though you have murdered him. If you look with lust on a woman, it is as though you have committed adultery. If someone sues you in court and takes your shirt, give him your coat as well. And the capstone? Do not love only those who love you, but love your enemies as well.

By now, the connections between mirror neurons and our Christian lives are quite clear. Since that day on a Galilean mountainside, we have known our marching orders. Christians are to love their neighbors as themselves. Yet the idea that we are to love our neighbors as ourselves can feel like an impossibly huge task. Is Jesus asking far more from his followers than they can possibly give? If slapped, must we really offer the other cheek also? This love often requires sacrifice and long-term commitment to the welfare of another. Sometimes we wonder if we really have it in us.

Yet Jesus' command is not the lofty expectation of a religious prodigy. It is the imperative of the One who knows our frame, who was present as we were formed in our mother's womb. His command only codifies our bodies' innate capability. As if reaching back before the fall, Jesus calls up the God-given abilities of his followers and commands that, for those walking in the Spirit, the law is now only the lowest common denominator. It is as if Jesus is saying, "You were made for more."

Though our attempts may be marred by sin, we have indeed been created for this purpose—to love our neighbors, even our enemies, as ourselves. Mirror neurons allow us to connect with others, decoding and understanding their emotions and actions in ways that can shape our relationships. We won't perfectly love our neighbors as ourselves, and despite our mirror neurons we'll likely always be baffled by other people, whose thoughts can be so different from ours. Yet we can at times understand our neighbors' needs before consciously thinking about them. And we can experience all the emotions felt by those among us. We feel their happiness, pain, curiosity, surprise, grief, excitement and more. This mimicry provides the foundation for empathy and compassion, key components for fulfilling Jesus' commands. We can see our neighbor no longer as other but as intimately connected to us, and the enactment of Jesus' commands becomes not a pipe dream but the joyful duty of the kingdom of God in our midst.

4

LIFE TOGETHER

BY THE MID-EIGHTEENTH CENTURY, the Methodist movement was growing rapidly in England. When local Methodists needed to pay off some debt used to take over a building, someone proposed forming the Methodist followers into societies and charging dues of a penny apiece. After a while, members of these societies formed smaller groups of classes, for instruction, and even smaller bands, which functioned as small groups. The bands, which American Methodist pioneer Francis Asbury called "little families of love," became the means by which the Methodists formed disciples.

These Methodist bands were not merely taught the right things to believe—though there was plenty of theological instruction. John Wesley preached and was well known for it—by the end of his life he had delivered more than forty thousand sermons. But he didn't assume that when his followers assented to Methodist theology they would immediately and strictly practice it in their lives. When he left the pulpit or the field where he was preaching, these small groups served as places in which people could practice his teaching.

Wesley understood that we need others and that the influence of those we surround ourselves with is as powerful a force—perhaps more so—than the most thunderous sermon. "Christianity is essentially a social religion," Wesley said, "and . . . to turn it into a solitary religion is indeed to destroy it." He clarified how important he felt was the context of our faith: Christianity, he said, "cannot subsist at all without society, without living and conversing with [others]."[1]

The Methodists succeeded as a movement in large part because they understood that it is through regular gatherings with intimate groups that discipleship happens. Because the Methodists believed in the perfectibility of people as followers of God, they needed this approach to train disciples. These groups "enriched and sustained" this new style of evangelical faith. "Though it is God only [who] changes hearts," Wesley said, "yet he generally doth it by man."[2]

Methodist bands were effective. A study of more than five hundred profiles of Methodists published in the denomination's early magazines has revealed that only a quarter of converts joined the movement as a result of preaching. "By far the majority needed the nurture of the society, classes and bands, and spent an average of 2.3 years in this nurturing process before experiencing what they identified as new birth."[3]

The bands were particularly effective on the frontier of America, where settlers often moved well before churches were in place, and where the initial pioneers were not likely to have been churchgoers. A frontier Kentucky woman, thinking her husband needed a good dose of religion, persuaded him to visit her Methodist class. First they prayed and sang hymns, and then they broke up into smaller groups. James Finley said, "I never heard more plain, simple, scriptural common sense, yet eloquent views of Christian experience in my life. . . . It was a time of profound and powerful feeling."[4] He ended the meeting in tears and firmly committed to his new faith.

Most contemporary churches utilize their own form of Wesley's little families of love. We call them small groups, cell groups, life groups or community groups. But whatever name we use, our intent is the same—to give churchgoers the opportunity for intimate relationships that promote the flourishing of their faith. In fact, it is commonly believed that the growth and maintenance of today's megachurches occurs only because these churches provide people with a way to connect with others in a small group. It's not enough to attend a weekend service with thousands of people. To get and stay connected, you must find your tribe. In his profile of Rick Warren and Saddleback Church, Malcolm Gladwell writes that the key to the church's success is its small groups. More important than prayer or worship, close relationships connect people to the church, to God and to the rest of their community. "Membership in a small group is a better predictor of whether people volunteer or give money than how often they attend church, whether they pray, whether they've had a deep religious experience, or whether they were raised in a Christian home," Gladwell writes.[5]

Furthermore, it isn't what you believe theologically that influences your behavior, it is who you are connected to. Princeton sociologist Robert Wuthnow says that in his research, "I was finding that if people say all the right things about being a believer but aren't involved in some kind of physical social setting that generates interaction, they are just not as likely to volunteer."[6] It isn't your decision for Christ that makes you act like a Christian but whom you invite for dinner on Wednesday nights.

These practices are not simply an effective way of doing church. They are rooted and flow forth from our very design. There is no creature on the planet quite as social as a human being. From the moment we are born, we seek to connect to others, and this biological need continues throughout our lives. We all want to belong to and with someone else.

Our Social Bodies

Around the world, people are gathering to cuddle. Not couples by a warm fire or a child in his father's lap: these people are strangers. When friends expressed a desire for nonsexual physical intimacy, relationship coaches Reid Mihalko and Marcia Baczynski founded Cuddle Party, a group where adults could simply enjoy snuggling. The popularity of these groups spread quickly, and in less than ten years cuddle parties cropped up around the world. Mihalko told the *Washington Post,* "We all want touch in our lives, but nobody's telling each other."[7]

Our need for touch is so strong that today people are willing to even cuddle with strangers to fulfill those needs. We all need the encouragement, comfort, support and care that a loving touch can provide. In fact, touch is vital to our functioning as social bodies, created by God to love and serve one another.

In an experiment, researchers tried to determine whether people could accurately convey a specific emotion through a five-second touch. Subjects were blindfolded, and then a stranger touched them on different parts of the body—the arm, face, head, hands, shoulders, trunk or back. The touchers attempted to convey a specific emotion: anger, fear, happiness, sadness, disgust, love, gratitude or sympathy. The blindfolded subject was then asked to identify the emotion or determine that there was no emotion conveyed. Chance would have suggested that subjects could have guessed correctly about 11 percent of the time. Yet subjects accurately interpreted the emotion of a touch between 50 and 78 percent of the time.[8]

Other research confirms these findings. One study found that subjects in the United States and Spain could accurately interpret one of twelve emotions conveyed by the touch of a stranger on the arm. They also found that observers could determine the emotion of a touch simply by watching it.[9] In both cases, accuracy was far better than chance, with accuracy ranging between 48 percent and 83 percent.[10]

How is it possible to feel someone's disgust in a fingertip placed on the arm? It turns out that our skin has two types of nerve receptors. One is used in manipulating objects, which we use to type, swing a hammer or sew a dress. But the other type of receptor is "connected to the core of our social brain," according to Louis Cozolino, a psychology professor at Pepperdine University, and "dedicated to communicative emotional touch." Cozolino writes, "Light touch and comfortable warmth lead to increases in oxytocin and endorphins that enhance social bonds through an association with a feeling of well-being. Touch also leads to mild sedation, decreases in blood pressure, and aids in autonomic regulation and cardiovascular health."[11]

Our connections to other people run far deeper than the skin, however. Researchers have discovered through studies of twins that a student's genes determined about half of the variation they found in the students' popularity. In other words, all the ways in which you have learned to be social, to be polite and friendly, all put together, are worth only about 54 percent of your ability to attract friends. The rest is determined by your genes. According to the authors of the study, "On average, a person with, say, five friends has a different genetic makeup than a person with one friend."[12]

But the study goes further. Genes equally affect where you stand among your friends. "Your genes affect not just how many friends you have but also whether you are located in the center or at the periphery of the network. On average, people located in central parts of the network have a different genetic makeup than those located at the periphery."[13]

While our genes affect the network of our friendships, our friends also affect us. Upon meeting someone, we immediately begin to synch ourselves with that person. David Brooks offers a compelling example of how quickly and easily we attune ourselves with others. "It took Muhammad Ali, who was just about as quick as anybody ever, 190 milliseconds to detect an opening in his opponent's defenses and begin throwing a punch into it. It takes the average college student 21 milliseconds to begin synchronizing her movement unconsciously with her friends."[14] When friends are talking in deep conversation, they begin to mimic each other's breathing patterns. People watching the conversation do the same, and the more they mimic the body language, the more perceptive they are about the conversation.[15]

Finally, this physical mimicry, as we saw in the last chapter, produces emotional synchronization. When a friend is happy, we mimic his smiles and the contraction of the muscles around the eyes that give us "crows' feet" in the corners of our eyes as we age. (Take a moment and smile only with your mouth. Now do it again so that the corners of your eyes scrunch up. Feel the difference?) We begin to mimic a person's happiness when we get our own "happy muscles" working. Once again, researchers are finding that the body is helping the mind to think: "The path of the signals is from the muscles (of the face) to the brain, rather than the more usual efferent pathway from the brain to the muscles."[16] This is why many telemarketers and others who sell over the phone are trained to smile. Though you can't see them, you will hear their cheerfulness.

Our Social Brains

Connections to other people are not merely regulated by our bodies' genes, nerves and muscles. These relationships also affect our brains, changing what we think and even *how* we think. If we seek to understand how the Methodist bands and today's small groups form disciples, then we need to look even further to how the people with whom we surround ourselves will actually change who we are.

Studies have shown that Easterners and Westerners perceive the world differently. People in the more communal cultures of Asia tend to focus on groups, while Westerners tend to see the individual. When shown the same picture, say of a school of fish, those in the East will respond to questions by describing the school and perhaps the relationships between the fish. Westerners, who tend to be more individualistic, focus on a single fish and describe it. In a number of tests like this, studies have confirmed that Western individualism shapes how we see the world around us. But that cultural emphasis on the individual changes more than how we perceive a picture or the objects we focus on in a painting. It also changes the way in which our brain works.

"When an American thinks about whether he is honest," summarizes a report on recent studies for the American Psychological Association, "his brain activity looks very different than when he thinks about whether another person is honest." Yet in brain images of Chinese thinking about their own and others' honesty, their brain activity appears to be identical in each case. Another study found that when Easterners viewed shapes of people in positions of "submission," such as the head hanging down, the reward circuitry—the brain's "feel-good system"—fired, giving a mildly good feeling, perhaps below the level of consciousness. In the United States, where dominance is valued, the reward circuitry fired when subjects viewed images of people in "dominant" positions, such as standing tall with their arms crossed.[17]

Studies like these show how cultural values can be embedded in our biology. Whether those values promote the good of others or only the good of self, they may be hardwired into our brains.

But our own experiences get hardwired as well to *produce* these fruits—or not to. Research among mammals shows that when raised without a father, animals develop neural connections at a slower rate and tend to have less control over their impulses. Humans are far more sensitive to these effects. Neural connection is related to intelligence, while controlling impulses is related to socially respectable behavior and fortitude in pursuing life goals. As neurologist David Eagleman writes, "Becoming socialized is nothing but developing [the neural] circuitry to squelch our basest impulses."[18]

There is another way in which our social connections are related to our intelligence. Brain researchers say that the size of our brain is perfectly predicted by the size of our social group. Living within a large group of people is an intellectually demanding task. We must understand a range of personalities and navigate the complex web of relationships among friends and family.

Anyone who has ever planned a party or arranged seats at a wedding understands this. *What will happen if we put these family members with those friends from work and this couple from church?* Or *We can't put Katie at a table with the Webbers!* Or *He's so loud the Millers will never have a chance to speak.*

The possible number of relationships between people grows exponentially the more people enter a social group. While there is one relationship between two people, there are ten among five people. "Humans are 'ultrasocial,' with skills ranging from language to abstract reasoning to empathy and insight that are adapted to a highly social environment," write researchers James Fowler and Nicholas Christakis.[19] This demands immense cognitive work.

By comparing the optimal group size of a number of different primate species, researcher Robin Dunbar showed how group size and brain size were directly correlated. He then predicted that humans' brain size would suggest our expected group size should be 150, which is the maximum size at which humans function together easily and without splintering.[20]

The Social Network

There is another way in which our relationships with other people affect us. It's clear that our friends, family and coworkers, and others with whom we directly relate, have powerful effects on who we are, the things we believe, our commitments to faith and family, our desires, and even how we perceive the world around us. In addition, people who are two and even three degrees removed from us can exert influence in our lives.

Our friends' friends can change who we are—even the kind of relationships our friends have with their friends. It makes a difference what kinds of relationships our family members have with one another, regardless of our individual relationship with each member. We are even affected by the structure of the social network we inhabit, whether we are lightly connected to a number of different and unconnected groups, for example, or deeply connected to just one or two groups.

One economist found that the likelihood of your becoming a parent dramatically increases in the two years after one of your siblings has a baby. The study of eight thousand families found that not only are you likely to start your family soon after your sibling has a baby, but you're likely to have more kids. In other words, if you'd planned to have two children by age thirty-five and your sister starts having children at twenty-five, you may end up having three children by thirty-two. The effects are similar in non-Western countries.[21]

There is a whole range of ways our friends and family and their friends and family influence us. We give away more money when our coworkers do—even when we don't know their giving habits. You gain in happiness by about 15 percent when your friend's friend is happy; that's about the same effect as for gaining eighty thousand dollars.[22] We will tend to lose weight when our friends' friends do. I have seen this personally after a friend introduced me to the workout room at the office. He got me going, and my coworkers saw me sweaty after lunch and started joining us.

If you are married, consider how you found your spouse. Finding a mate is just one way our network affects us, but it provides a way to look at the structure of that network. The size of our network matters. The more friends and family (who can introduce us to their friends) we have, the more potential spouses we have the opportunity to meet. But its structure also matters, as does where we stand in that network. If we are loosely connected to a number of people, our connections are constantly shifting, and our friends behave similarly in their own networks. Thus we are very likely to come across a number of people to whom we might be attracted. On the other hand, if we are tightly bonded to just a few people (even within a large network) and they are tightly linked to others with little flow, our chances of finding a spouse diminish. Even through dating websites that offer varying levels of anonymity, some people who eventually marry may discover a previous loose connection to each other.

We need both strong and loose ties to others, not only in our personal lives but also economically. The financial and innovative engines of cities have been linked to the many loose ties they foster. People come across new ideas and spread them quickly. They move from job to job, picking up new skills and sharing them with new companies. At the same time, people need some stability in order to get to know those with whom they are working with and understand their strengths and weaknesses.

Brian Uzzi, a professor at Northwestern University, studied the networks of those who put on Broadway musicals. He found that the ideal network for success was one with lots of tight cliques with connections between them. When people worked together too often, they lost their creative edge, unable to use new ideas. On the other hand, when people hadn't worked together enough, they didn't know how to work together, and their shows flopped. Success depended on a tight core group with some fresh blood.[23]

A wide variety of connections open new worlds to us, give us new opportunities and expose us to different kinds of people with unique tastes and ideas. If you are job hunting or looking for a new doctor, seeking out a church or a good friend, the possibilities open to you through your acquaintances, coworkers and casual friendships can help you discover what you need. Further, broad and shallow connections are especially useful because they give us increased opportunities to develop what we *most* need: deep and lasting relationships. Knowing others and being known by them, supporting and caring for others and receiving that same support, are essential for our happiness.

Belonging, Then Believing

Our relationships—with family, friends, coworkers, neighbors—are deeply related to our faith. In their studies of religion, sociologists Rodney Stark and Roger Finke write that social connections have a profound effect on the strength of church groups and denominations. Smaller churches tend to grow the fastest, they say, because the relationships between members are dense. Close relationships among members tend to draw outsiders in as well as keep current members a part of the group.

As a church grows, the connections between members tend to become diffuse, commitment declines, and growth ebbs. Members of larger churches, because they do not have strong connections to other members, usually have more relationships outside the church. Because of that, they also seek to push the church to become more like the outside society, and as the church moves toward accommodation with society it loses its reason for being. Commitment declines and so does membership.[24] All this unless the larger church can harness the power of relationships to keep members committed to their faith and to one another.

Where I live, on the West Coast, most churches tend to be small and to have little influence in the culture. Stark and Finke explain, "A major reason for the lack of church membership in the West is high rates of mobility, which decrease the ability of all voluntary organizations, not just churches, to maintain membership. That is, people move so often that they lack the social ties needed to affiliate with churches."[25]

To address this problem, one of the most effective church-planting networks in the United States began in Tacoma, Washington, by using a method of developing intensive community in neighborhoods. Soma Communities fosters deep and intense relationships by teaching church planters to get closely involved in their neighborhoods, opening their homes to neighbors, gathering friends together on a regular basis, and forming "missional communities" focused on discovering and meeting the needs of neighbors and the community.

It is these relational bonds that make someone unfamiliar with Christianity want to try it out. Rick Richardson, who directs the evangelism and leadership program at Wheaton College Graduate School, argues that "belonging comes before believing." He contrasts older methods of evangelism that focused on asking individuals to make a set of commitments. Today, asserts Richardson, presenting four spiritual laws and inviting people to make decisions for Christ is less effective. "Evangelism is about helping people belong so that they can come to believe. So our communities need to be places where people can connect before they have to commit."[26] The idea is held up by social science research showing that converts tend to sign on to a new faith only after their social ties become stronger to those in the new faith than to others outside it. "This often occurs before a convert knows much about what the group believes."[27]

Gerald Sittser notes that the early church didn't grow through public displays, rallies or debates with reigning intellectuals. Yet the growth of the early church was phenomenal—simple. "Christians bartered in the same markets, drew water from the same wells. . . . The church thus attracted outsiders through natural networks." Sittser says this infuriated the church's opponents. The Christians were "able to convince only the foolish, dishonorable and stupid, and only slaves, women and little children," complained the philosopher Celsus. They converted people one at a time. "In private houses also we see wool-workers, cobblers, laundry-workers, and the most bucolic yokels, who would not dare to say anything at all in front of their elders and more intelligent masters," Celsus wrote. While their "betters" fumed, the Christians' message was received in these private settings where people offered one-on-one friendship, care and support.[28]

Acts 16 tells us how Paul and his companions settled at the edge of a river in an area where they "supposed there was a place of prayer." A group of women was assembled there, among them a purple cloth seller named Lydia. In the midst of this group of women—probably friends—Lydia responded to the gospel. Acts tells us that she was a "worshiper of God" though she had not yet heard Jesus' gospel; she had at least the rudimentary knowledge to fit into the group, and probably after months of visiting with these women, her heart was primed to respond. Lydia was baptized and immediately began to reach out to others, offering hospitality to Paul and other believers.

We, with Lydia, were designed to connect deeply with God. As we seek to share the gospel with those around us, we cannot discount the ways in which our relationships may provide a safe space for another person to hear and embrace the good news. In different ways we are primed to believe in God and to connect to other people from the moment of our birth. Those two connections are closely related. A relationship with another person may be the catalyst that draws him or her into relationship with God himself.

5

WIRED FOR INTIMACY

Two weeks after I experienced a radical spiritual awakening in my early twenties, I met the woman who would become my wife. My experience of God had already begun to affect my social life, and as I look back, Clarissa's arrival on the scene is woven seamlessly into the story of my reborn love for God.

I was already high on God when I arrived at the wedding of two college friends that warm May evening. After what had been a long dry spell, I once again craved time in prayer and fellowship with other believers. My brain was afire with passion for God, and my heart was ready to engage in spiritual relationships with others. While I wasn't looking for a spouse, I can see now how my renewed spiritual life was changing the way I connected with others. So it is no wonder that while walking up a flight of stairs to the sanctuary, I was drawn to stop and talk to the beautiful brown-eyed girl walking in the other direction.

We sat together during the ceremony and found ourselves surprisingly delighted to both be assigned to the "singles table" at the reception. I'd like to thank the table of loosely related acquaintances who jabbered the night away, providing me the opportunity to monopolize the attentions of the lovely guest seated beside me. The following day, when she joined the singles table for an excursion to

Boston, I was thrilled. In the context of that group, we were already forming the connections that would blossom into love.

In the weeks and months that followed, we emailed—since we lived far apart—writing lengthy epistles of observations and commentary on events of the day. I've saved nearly two hundred emails from the first few months we knew each other, and these are only the longer ones. We talked on the phone for hours and hours. Today I can't imagine making a phone call that would last for thirty minutes, and Clarissa generally dislikes making *any* phone call. But as we fell in love, we desired each other's company. Like any couple in love, we thought constantly about each other, pined away during our time apart.

In the span of two weeks one spring, I had become obsessed with two things: God and this beautiful, spirited girl. After six months, she came for a visit, and I determined I'd had enough. I would ask Clarissa to be my bride. No more waiting for her calls. No more checking and double-checking for new emails. No more listless pining. (I had done my fair share.) I wanted to be with her forever. So on a chilly autumn night, I knelt beside a river and asked Clarissa to be my wife. That day she developed a cold, and later she lost her voice. I like to think she was speechless with joy.

If You Knew What You Were In For

Not long before Clarissa and I were married, my father gave me a cryptic admonition. "If you knew what you were getting into, Rob," he said, "you wouldn't do it." An odd remark, to be sure, from a happily married man to his son on the threshold of marital bliss.

It was a strange thing to say, but it was how Dad talked about his relationship with God as well. At a point in his early twenties he had met God, as I did, in a sudden and dramatic way. It changed his life. Dad's early "romance" with God had been thrilling, but the realization that a long-term spiritual relationship required work, effort and sacrifice had come as a sobering—and maturing—experience. He would use the same joking phrase to describe his marriage and spiritual experiences: "You tricked me!" For Dad's relationship with God to continue in a meaningful way, he would have to become a disciple of Jesus and put the needs of others before his own. It would mean recognizing his selfishness and putting that aside. It would mean taking time away from watching sports or politics on television and spending time in prayer. As his love for the Lord grew, Dad found delight in those things that were difficult, seeing now that they were life-giving. His reasons for staying on with the Lord weren't necessarily the things that had attracted him in the first place.

I could not know what kind of work would be required of me as I set out on married life, but Dad assured me it would be worth it. As I was soon to find, Dad was right. Both in my spiritual life and in my marriage, the romance would come and go. If I were to depend on those feelings, I would be lost when they ebbed. But I could not think myself into love for God any more than I could think myself into love for Clarissa. The initial infatuation positioned me to be willing to make the dramatic changes that true attachment and real love would require.

We often think of marriage as a private relationship, reflecting only the personalities of the two individuals involved. The Bible, however, describes marriage as a uniquely corporate relationship. It is at once about a husband and wife and about Christ and the church, an unparalleled picture of what our life with God can be. As we discover how God has designed us for love and service, the image of marriage allows us to see this design at its most intimate level.

The biology of love illuminates this kind of obsession, a common mark of courtship. We focus on the object of our love, even giving it our full attention to the detriment of our health, our sleep, our diet. We pine for our beloved. As the poetry of Song of Songs declares:

> Restless night after night in my bed,
>> I longed and looked for my soul's true love;
> I searched for him
>> but I could not find him
> I will get up now and search the city,
>> wander up and down streets and plazas;
> I will look for my soul's true love.
>> I searched for him, but I could not find him. . . .
> Not long after I left them,
>> I found him—I found my soul's true love.
> I pulled him to me and would not let him go. (Song of Songs
>> 3:1-2, 4 *The Voice*)

These lines perfectly describe the first half of the biology of love: romance. The second half, attachment, keeps couples together over the years. Romance involves falling in love; attachment is born of the hard work of knitting two lives together. While romance may be fun and exciting, it leads nowhere if it doesn't culminate in attachment. Attachment often comes with more difficulty and forces us to learn to put the needs of others before our own, but it is the basis for a meaningful life.

Wired for Romance

There may be few things more unromantic than gathering a group of highly passionate, infatuated college students in order to shove their heads inside a brain scanner and decode the thoughts of love. In other experiments, researchers have taken the same approach with couples who have spent decades together. Pull Grandma and Grandpa off their rockers, put them into an fMRI machine, and figure out why they still give each other that special smile.

The science of love splits our romantic affections in half. First comes the head-over-heels stage in which we fall madly in love. This is the point where we become addicted to love. Chemically, this stage of wild passion is like a drug addiction. We forgo sleep and food because we can think of little else than the person we are drawn to. But, as with any drug, our bodies build up a tolerance, and each hit has a weaker effect. As our obsessive love matures, the biology of love changes from passion to attachment. The chemicals involved change from producing attention and the pursuit of a goal into those neuropeptides involved in bonding and cuddling and nurturing. Finally, this bonding and attachment chemical loosens our neurological connections, changing who we are and reshaping us into people attuned to the loves we have chosen.

Researchers have found that dopamine is related to lovers' need to be in touch constantly. They often say that for the brain, falling in love is similar to a hit of cocaine. "Elevated levels of dopamine in the brain produce extremely focused attention, as well as unwavering motivation and goal-directed behaviors."[1] Another trait of dopamine—and another feature that makes romantic desire similar to a cocaine rush—is that it produces a powerful feeling of elation or ecstasy. Two lovers experience a sense of excitement that overflows to the rest of their lives; when looking back on that period of their lives, the lovers recall a magical time in which everything was bathed in an enchanted glow.

All of these are wonderful feelings. We like having them and want more. Naturally, then, another effect of dopamine is a craving for more and a dependency on the beloved to produce those feelings again. The turmoil that separated lovers feel is due in part to the brain's production of more dopamine when the "cocaine rush" of being with the beloved is delayed. Desire for the absent fruit causes greater desire for it and more intense anxiety until that fruit is tasted.

In fact, some researchers prefer not to think of love itself as a feeling or an emotion but rather as a "motivational state" that leads us to pursue the feelings of euphoria we get as we fall in love. "A person in love has the keenest possible ambition to achieve a goal," says David Brooks. "A person in love is in a state of need."[2] The parts of our brain that produce this state are also those parts that are involved in the most fundamental actions of existence, such as muscle memory enabling us to talk or run without conscious thought about how to do so.[3] Love is one of our most basic needs.

Laboratory scientists will measure the addictive power of a chemical by making a rat push a bar to get a drop of it. Depending on the substance, the rat may do nothing but push the bar for more and more, forgoing anything else. They've found dopamine has that effect. When we fall in love, we are like those rats, pumping the bar for more and more of our beloved.

Bonded

But love is not merely passionate pursuit. Scientists who write about love always talk about the prairie vole. It is a furry rodent, like a little gerbil, and lives in the grasslands between the Rocky Mountains and the Appalachians. Unlike other rodents, and even other voles, the prairie vole is monogamous. Following a twenty-four-hour period of mating, the male vole will never leave the female. Even if she dies, he will not seek another mate.

What makes this behavior so interesting to scientists is that the female prairie vole's monogamy can be turned off by removal of the chemical oxytocin, and the male's turned off by blocking a similar chemical called vasopressin. Shut off the oxytocin, and the cuddly, sensitive vole turns into a philanderer.[4]

Oxytocin is involved in all human bonding, producing the warm feelings we have after a night with close friends or a relaxing massage, or that a mother has when nursing her baby. All of the "goal-oriented behavior" of romantic love—the passionate pursuit of our beloved to the exclusion of all else—creates the perfect conditions for oxytocin's takeover of the neural system. The "cocaine rush" of falling in love transitions to the warm cuddles of attachment.

It is no wonder, then, that so many couples choose 1 Corinthians 13 to be read at their weddings. Though this passage on love is directed to a church congregation, its description of the connecting qualities of love is second to none. The apostle Paul writes,

> Love is patient, love is kind. It does not envy, it does not boast, it is not proud. It does not dishonor others, it is not self-seeking, it is not easily angered, it keeps no record of wrongs. Love does not delight in evil but rejoices with the truth. It always protects, always trusts, always hopes, always perseveres. (1 Cor 13:4-7)

All these things are related to oxytocin. When researchers try to boil down the recipe for successful marriages, they are unable to improve on this passage. Happy couples, according to one group of researchers, "idealized their partners; they overestimated their partner's virtues . . . and underestimated their faults."[5] They give of themselves over and over again for years and years. It is oxytocin that aids our transition from an individual fulfilling our own desires, to a lover ambitiously pursuing another, to a companion for life who seeks the good of someone else. Oxytocin makes it happen. Yet oxytocin, of course, is not a marriage chemical. It appears anywhere close, healthy relationships exist. You don't need to say "I do" in order to give of yourself over and over to another person or people, to rejoice with the truth, protect, trust, hope and persevere. Commitment to work for the best in other people is a part of the journey toward holiness that anyone should pursue.

Paul's formula of love has positive and negative components, and oxytocin is related to each. Love is patient and kind; it rejoices and perseveres. But dealing with envy and anger is also necessary for lifetime bonding. The love chemicals, dopamine and oxytocin, not only contribute to positive feelings but also shut down the lovers' ability to think negatively. UC Berkeley researcher Dacher Keltner writes that "romantic love deactivates threat detection regions of the brain—the right prefrontal cortical regions and the amygdala."[6] (Perhaps this is also why someone abused by a lover may too quickly try to think the best of that person.)

Oxytocin also reduces the activity of brain regions associated with stress. Oxytocin and its sister attachment chemical vasopressin are both dumped into the brain during orgasm, creating the powerful sense of connection during those moments and maintaining or increasing overall feelings of bonding. Sex, then, isn't just fun. The chemical components make us willing and able to give of ourselves for the sake of the other person.

These romance chemicals have one other feature, in addition to helping us bond with those we love. They shake up the neurological connections in our brains. As our neurons fire together, they "wire together." This makes our brain more efficient by laying down a pathway for a brain process that will be repeated over and over again. We don't easily disrupt these neural pathways.

Bonding to another person, however, requires the undoing of a number of brain pathways. Oxytocin, according to some scientists, is an "amnestic hormone." It allows us to *unlearn* behavior. The chemical "melts down existing neuronal connections that underlie existing attachments, so new attachments can be formed." Oxytocin doesn't just help us to be patient and kind. It doesn't simply reduce our tendencies toward pride and boastfulness. We are still who we are, but the attachment chemicals enable us to undo any behaviors and attitudes that would prevent us from fully bonding and attaching to those we love.

In one sense, this is the greatest miracle that sex produces, though certainly procreation is miraculous as well. In the sexual experience we are able to *change who we are,* turning away from being individuals focused on our own desires, our own ideas and our own gratification. In sexual love, we become new people as we emerge as "one flesh" from the union we have chosen.

The biology of love first produces that remarkable and overwhelming desire for another person. But the desire is still to fulfill our own longing. Then we begin to bond. Like two atoms, fully stable and independent, we attach, and our electrons begin swirling around two different nuclei. Our edges become fuzzy, sometimes part of ourselves, other times part of the beloved. We unlearn what makes us individuals, and we learn what makes us "us."

Marriage to God

Throughout the Bible and church history, the relationship between human beings and God is compared to that of a husband and wife or two lovers in pursuit of one another. God compares his love for the creatures he created to the most intimate, passionate and consuming of human relationships. God tells Jeremiah of his love for

Israel, "I have loved you with an everlasting love; I have drawn you
with unfailing kindness" (Jer 31:3). He tells Isaiah, "For your Maker
is your husband" (54:5), and "As a bridegroom rejoices over his
bride, so will your God rejoice over you" (62:5).

Perhaps the most provocative example of how God seems to
view his relationship with human beings is in Hosea. God tells the
prophet to "marry a promiscuous woman" in order to illustrate the
way Israel has treated God. Hosea marries a woman named Gomer,
and they have children. But Gomer never gives up her other lovers,
and God tells Hosea this is how Israel's own promiscuity, worshiping other gods, makes him feel.

The motif of God as a husband continues until the very end of
the Bible. In the book of Revelation, in a profusion of metaphors,
John announces the completion of God's redemption process. He
watches a city descending from heaven—the church "prepared as
a bride beautifully dressed for her husband" (Rev 21:2). The angel
says, "Come, I will show you the bride, the wife of the Lamb" (21:9).

Describing the ecstasies of the spiritual life, Christian saints also
have envisioned their relationship with God in terms of a lover. Consider Bernard of Clairvaux. He was no solitary mystic, contem-
plating alone in his cell the wonders of divine unification. Instead,
he was a worldly-wise leader, crusader and adviser to princes.
Bernard founded seventy monasteries; he wrote the rule for the new
religious order of the Knights Templar, who were devoted to spiritual service and the military defense of Christendom. Through his
wide traveling and preaching he united Europe to respond to Muslim
advances during the Second Crusade. Bernard's commitment to the
Crusades ("Fly then to arms; let a holy rage animate you in the fight,"
he said in a sermon)[7] also shows us that a feeling of spiritual union
with God does not necessarily raise us above the sins of our age.

Still, Bernard spoke movingly of God as his lover. "The Word, the Bridegroom," he writes, "several times has come in unto me. . . . Through the renewing and refashioning of the spirit of my mind, that is, of my inner man, I perceived in some measure His excellent beauty; and from gazing upon all these things together I was filled with awe at His abundant greatness." Bernard writes, "This is the marriage-contract of a truly spiritual and holy union: no, contract is too weak a description; it is an embrace."[8]

Language similar to Bernard's can be found among many other medieval mystics, but it had antecedents in early church history, and its echoes reverberate today. In a study of the prayer practices of members of Vineyard churches, women were quoted as imagining having a date with God, who would show up as a real person to whom they can talk about the most mundane or the most intimate issues. Researcher T. M. Luhrmann writes, "The women would set aside the night, and they imagined it romantically: it was a 'date.' They might pick up dinner or set out a plate at the table, and they imagined their way through the evening talking to God, cuddling with God, and basking in God's attention."[9]

Language of "lover," "husband" or even "boyfriend" is common and consistent across centuries of religious experience. Some people may feel uncomfortable with the use of this imagery for God today. Perhaps this is because we tend to relate to God as someone far more remote. Or maybe the images of teen romance in pop songs simply don't translate well in contemporary worship music, in which such images are employed to address God. Nevertheless, human beings from biblical times to today have related to God as a lover.

The analogy isn't simply an attempt to compare two intense kinds of relationships. We use this language of love and union because that's how it *feels* to be absorbed in our experience of God. The practice of knowing God in prayer, in obedience, in the pursuit of holiness feels like that of marriage. We are first enraptured by the experience of God. When the initial passion subsides, our love deepens toward attachment. We submit our wills to the needs of another and find a deep joy and purpose, and help in our times of need. In the love of God or in a marriage, we replicate and share the love we experience with others. And we can still discover deep, intense and passionate moments of overwhelming joy and union that spur us toward a fuller submission and greater sense of being known and loved.

Marriage, of course, is not a requirement for holiness. There are paths of discipleship for single people, ways to pursue God, that are typically not available to a married couple and that the apostle Paul argues are even better than marriage. And there are other, non-sexual forms of love and union available to people called to different forms of relationships. Yet marriage stands as an important picture of the possibilities of intimacy in our spiritual lives.

Wired for Destruction

The science of attachment shows us that love potion is real. Our bodies make chemicals powerful enough for us to be, in a sense, fatally attracted to another person. As with the love potions in fairytales, there is a dark side. The long, slow change that occurs in us through marriage and attachment can be short-circuited.

Over the last two decades, pornography escaped from behind the counters of shady shops in out-of-the-way areas to run free in accessible, even unavoidable, depravity. Its pervasive and widespread use has been called an epidemic, even where religious objections do not hold sway. The government of Iceland is considering a wholesale ban on Internet porn.[10] The government in the United Kingdom is demanding it.[11] Parents in England have been disturbed by the degree to which schoolboys are pressuring girls to enact what they view online.

Porn is the fourth most common reason people use the Internet, and it accounts for 25 percent of video rentals. Most of the time people are somewhat innocently hooked. A fun, but sexualized, video attracts a user toward more sexual images. Eventually he or she seeks out more sexual images and later certain kinds of pornographic ones. Soon pornography wields an addictive force in the life of its user. In fact, in one survey, 80 percent of respondents said their relationships or their jobs were currently at risk because of their online pornography habits.[12]

Pornography is destructive particularly because of the way it addicts the brain by hijacking the chemical process that is supposed to attach us to another person. People will spend more and more time on it, needing more time and greater stimulation in order to achieve the same rush. That time, which to an average user amounts to two hours per week and can be more than eleven hours for someone considered addicted, can disrupt relationships and responsibilities. But pornography's destructiveness is not due simply to the amount of time people spend using it. It is a betrayal of one's relationships, an effort to achieve intimacy without attending to the needs of another person. This false relationship has immediate consequences for our real relationships, especially for that person whom we have promised to have and to hold.

Any addictive drug works by simulating and enhancing the body's normal functions. Cocaine and heroin, for example, mimic the brain's "feel-good" chemicals like dopamine. The drugs give an overwhelming feeling that the neurochemical would normally provide in more modest doses. Pornography works in a similar way. Triggering the normal visual cues and mild dopamine rush that come with sexual thoughts, porn then offers an easy way to load up on the rush of neurochemicals that comes with orgasm. Psychiatrist and author Norman Doidge writes, "By hijacking our dopamine system, addictive substances give us pleasure without our having to work for it."[13]

The inordinate and unnatural measure of these chemicals enables the rewiring of the brain. The rush of dopamine that comes with orgasm is supposed to help us bond with the person we love. It feels great, but it also enables the brain to rewire, allowing us to become more attuned to the person with whom we are making love. When the orgasm comes after a session of looking at pictures or videos of other kinds of sexual scenes, the viewer actually rewires his sexual appetite. Counselors of porn addicts say their patients lose the ability to enjoy a human partner. At the same time, the viewer must go deeper and longer into his or her habit in order to achieve the same dopamine rush.

Doidge calls our culture's pornography addiction an epidemic. He has treated addicted men who paradoxically hate and despise their addiction but can't stay away. Porn, he says, excites but doesn't satisfy. It easily produces cravings but also tolerance to the drug. "The men at their computers looking at porn," he writes, "had been seduced into pornographic training sessions that met all the conditions required for plastic change of brain maps." As their pathways for sexual experience changed, men would stop finding their wives attractive. While sex within marriage promotes greater attachment to one's spouse and happiness over a lifetime, porn causes relational withdrawal and warps our sexual capacities.[14]

For a compassionate, scientific and practical book for Christians on getting free of pornography, see Wheaton College professor William Struthers's book *Wired for Intimacy: How Pornography Hijacks the Male Brain* (Downers Grove, IL: InterVarsity Press, 2009).

Sexual Healing

Dan had kept his pornography addiction a secret for more than ten years of his marriage, but one night he finally confessed to his wife.[15] A friend of his had confessed his own addiction, and now Dan could no longer keep his guilt under wraps.

Dan's confession nearly destroyed his marriage. Learning of the years of mental infidelity crushed his wife's trust. His spiritual life needed a complete and honest overhaul. Through professional therapy and honest accountability with his wife and friends, Dan is working to overcome his addiction. In fact, he told me giving up pornography turned out to be the easy part. The harder work, he found, was confronting his more fundamental impulses toward selfishness, which were not limited to his computer use. Months of agonizing relational repair and years of rebuilding trust would be needed to rewire his brain.

It is widely accepted that there is a critical period of brain formation in early childhood that affects our sexuality for the rest of our lives. In the same way that the brain is designed to quickly learn language during childhood, it also appears there is a formation period—before adolescence—in which our brains take on their sexual shape. This is why our adult loves may reflect our childhood relationships with our parents. There are no hard-and-fast rules. However, Doidge says, "if the parent is warm, gentle, and reliable, the child will frequently develop a taste for that kind of relationship later on; if the parent is disengaged, cool, distant, self-involved, angry, ambivalent, or erratic, the child may seek out an adult mate who has similar tendencies."[16] Abuse or early sexual experiences during this critical period can have damaging effects that last a lifetime.

However, in many cases, like Dan's, unhealthy patterns can be consciously confronted and the brain rewired even in adulthood. When the mind is consciously directed toward healthy loves, the oxytocin and dopamine can loosen up those neural pathways and allow new ones to be formed. It is hard work, to be sure, but it is not impossible. We cannot erase the past and begin again with a clean slate. But we can redirect our brains toward patterns that promote health and right living.

Today Dan actively pursues healthy relationships with his wife, family and friends. He proactively admits his weakness, seeking to help others who have struggled with the same addiction. Dan isn't a new person, but he is a much healthier version of himself—mentally and spiritually. And his story of returning to his true love echoes the biblical one.

While God refers to himself as his people's lover, he passionately pursues them even when they have turned elsewhere. In Hosea, God says that he is like the man married to a woman with lovers all over town. Yet he vows to win her back. "Therefore I am now going to allure her," he says; "I will lead her into the wilderness and speak tenderly to her." And God boldly envisions his lover as faithful: "'In that day,' declares the LORD, 'you will call me "my husband"'" (Hos 2:14, 16).

When we consider how fraught with pain our sexuality can be, it is a wonder that God chose the intimacy of the marriage relationship as the picture of his love for us. We possess the capacity to passionately connect and grievously err. Yet it is in this picture that we see the greatest expression of the gospel, as "love to the loveless shown, that they might lovely be."[17]

6

STRENGTH
IN WEAKNESS

On a beautiful sunny July day, six weeks after giving birth to our fourth child, Clarissa sat nursing on our sofa and suddenly a wave of heat rushed through her. *I can barely breathe. I think I'm going to pass out.* She thought. *No. Am I having a heart attack? My chest is tight. My heart is pounding. I'm going to die. I'll slump to the ground, a crying newborn in my arms, the kids playing wildly around me, and nobody will know until Rob walks in the door at six o'clock. I'm going to die, and there is no one here to save me.*

Over the next few days, she began having multiple panic attacks. Sometimes they would cascade—one, two, three on top of each other in the space of an hour. Respite for an hour or so and then more. Adrenaline would rush through her body, a feeling so strong she'd have to shake her arms to try to make it go away. And she was frantic and terrified—*I can't be alone with my kids. I'm going to die.*

Within a week, Clarissa's body was so fatigued that she could barely sit up. The heart-rate increase that accompanied a simple walk to the bathroom would prompt a panic attack. She lost bowel control. She lost eight pounds in a week. And she worried incessantly—about our baby dying, about herself dying, about losing her mind. We would lie in bed at night, Clarissa nursing our daughter and desperately drinking in her newborn smell, and chant, "Be still. Be still." But her postpartum body refused to obey.[1]

Clarissa's rapidly deteriorating health was frightening to watch. The panic attacks completely depleted her energy, and for the next ten weeks she was nearly an invalid. We feared she was losing her mind. Her midwife urged us to find help immediately, and Clarissa visited myriad health care providers looking for something that would "fix" her body. Diagnosed with postpartum anxiety she was told to sleep more. Nurse more. Drink more water. Exercise. Blow into a bag. Eat protein. Avoid chocolate. Exorcise guilt. Create more "me time." Meditate. Pray. She was given medications that knocked her out, made her hallucinate and gave her infections. Sometimes the doctors and pharmacist contradicted each other. *Take this; no, wait, you can't. Well, it probably won't affect your nursing baby.* We were drowning in expert advice.

Four months after getting sick, under the direction of a psychiatrist and naturopathic doctor, Clarissa stopped all medication to pursue a more natural path to recovery. The naturopath ordered a test to measure brain chemicals and found that Clarissa had extremely low levels of nearly every one measured. She prescribed a rigorous regime of supplements to support the brain's own work of producing GABA, serotonin, dopamine and other amino acids, along with weekly acupuncture to promote healing. It would be a long road to recovery, she warned us, and we must accept the new normal of living with this disorder. More than two years later, we see that she was right.

Clarissa's illness occurred about halfway through my writing of this book, while I was immersing myself in research about the glorious design of our bodies. The contradiction between what we were experiencing and what I was writing was impossible to avoid. How could I stand in awe of God's glorious design for our bodies when things could go so badly wrong? How could our celebration of a birth become so marred by mental illness?

Seeing her so sick rattled my belief in this project. As she struggled to make spiritual sense of her experience, I had to question whether we really *are* biologically equipped to commune with God. I realized in a new and personal way that our mental condition is fragile, our grasp on reality tenuous. How could I assert with any confidence that we are so wonderfully designed and capable of deep connections with others and with God when our sanity seemed entirely dependent on a few grams of serotonin in the brain?

And yet in the sorrowful experience of mental illness we also have connected deeply with Jesus, the God who suffers the pain of a broken creation with us. Even with a malfunctioning brain, there has been peace and comfort, though not perfect healing. More important, we have become better attuned to respond to the sufferings of others. It is there—where suffering turns to compassion—that the questions provoked by suffering can find resolution.

I work for an organization that confronts this broken world every day. A typhoon rips through the Philippines, killing thousands, and leaving millions homeless, jobless and without food and water. In the absence of proper sanitation facilities and clean water, disease spreads and more people die. A tsunami hits Japan and causes a nuclear disaster. Rain fails to fall in Africa for years at a time. Livestock die, water runs out, crops fail. Mothers carry their babies to find help and food, but eventually, weak from hunger, they set them under a tree hoping someone else might care for them. An earthquake levels the most populous city in Haiti, the country least equipped—being the poorest in the Western Hemisphere—to respond to the disaster.

The world's brokenness exists not just on the five o'clock news but intimately, in our own bodies, as well. Disability, disease and death all reflect that the world is not as it should be. I spent years as a hospice volunteer, and with each patient I visited, the sorrow of death never lessened. Suffering may be a normal part of life, but that doesn't mean we must feel comfortable in a world of illness and death. I visited Parkinson's patients, who suffer from the body's inability to produce enough dopamine for the brain. I visited Alzheimer's patients, who suffer from plaque formations in the brain that prevent it from working correctly. As much as we understand these illnesses, their effects on people we know and love are proof enough that the world's brokenness has taken hold in our very cells.

The cracks in our broken world run even deeper than disease and natural disasters, however. Much of the suffering we experience comes from hopes dashed, people who fail us and our own failures. Many Christians have argued that we experience suffering because people are free to act in harmful ways. Yet as we study how profoundly our minds are connected to the physical workings of our brains, we can see that we may not be as free as we think. Even our free will is subject to a fallen creation.

If we are to consider how we may respond to bodily suffering, we must acknowledge that in a cosmic sense all is deeply and devastatingly broken. We must recognize that this brokenness exists in us however healthy we may appear on the outside. Even the chemical makeup and the physical functioning of our brains affect our thoughts, which then drive our actions for good or evil. This realization need not plunge us into despondency. Rather, this honest accounting of our condition can be the gateway through which we release the guilt that so often accompanies suffering. We can embrace our weakness, and we can find purpose to serve others with the strength given us from the God who offers us comfort and wholeness.

Beginning to Heal from the Inside Out

Wouldn't it be wonderful if we could choose to be healed—if we could choose to avoid all thoughts and behaviors that cause suffering to ourselves and others? Unfortunately, the effects of the curse run deep. We are shaped by our biology, our history and our environment in ways outside our control. These forces can drive our behaviors in ways that lead to our suffering and the suffering of others.

Many Christians argue that we choose to inflict suffering on ourselves and others when we act in opposition to God. Such an argument looks exclusively to the Bible's image of sin as a legal infraction. In the apostle Paul's discussion of sin and death and judgment, he uses legal images of lawbreaking and punishment. "All who sin under the law will be judged by the law. For it is not those who hear the law who are righteous in God's sight, but it is those who obey the law who will be declared righteous" (Rom 2:12-13). Those who are not Jews, and not subject to the law of Moses, Paul says, are still subject to those laws evident in creation. When they obey God's law on their own, they merely prove that the law is right.

This line of reasoning is true, but when it comes to our own choices it is not the whole story. Paul also recognizes how helpless he is to simply choose to obey the law. "Although I want to do good, evil is right there with me. For in my inner being I delight in God's law; but I see another law at work in me, waging war against the law of my mind and making me a prisoner of the law of sin at work within me" (Rom 7:21-23).

Augustine of Hippo, the fourth-century bishop and author of *The Confessions*, wrestled with the same inability to choose what he knew he ought to. After years of attempting to live an ideal life, first in the Gnostic sect of the Manichees, then as a Platonist philosopher and finally as a Christian, he became a priest and a bishop and discovered that none of his congregants had any better mastery over their choices. He writes, "The enemy held fast my will, and had made of it a chain, and had bound me tight with it. For out of the perverse will came lust, and the service of lust ended in habit, and habit, not resisted, became necessity. By these links, as it were, forged together—which is why I called it 'a chain'—a hard bondage held me in slavery."[6]

This bondage is, in large part, enslavement to the broken creation at work in our own biology. As we seek to accept our suffering, we must release its power to God and take on our new identity as broken people being restored by a loving God. This is the power of the gift of grace. Many times releasing guilt is a first step toward accepting our suffering and redeeming it.

As soldiers return from war, they carry with them a major psychological complication—their sense of guilt. Many worry whether God will accept them because of their actions in battle. Nancy Sherman, a professor at Georgetown University, interviewed dozens of veterans and found that a major part of the mental trauma they experience is due to guilt. "Individuals can feel guilty about actions for which they are not at fault, yet they hold themselves responsible."[7] Sherman tells the story of one D-Day soldier who landed on the beach in Normandy and felt terrible guilt decades

later for taking the gun of a killed comrade. It was an entirely jus-
tified action but still violated his sense of dignity. When it comes to
killing, the sense of moral guilt is much greater even when actions
are compelled by necessity and justifiable.

That's why Paul's legal answer is essential. Jesus paid the price for
our sins. Part of our suffering in this world is that we have taken
part in and perpetuated its brokenness. Even if a court of law
wouldn't hold us responsible (the tumor made me do it!), we can
still feel morally guilty about the ways our suffering affects others
and us. Yet we are set free by Jesus' death and resurrection, which
atone for our sins. With this legal freedom and the work of the
Spirit, the chains that once held us are broken.

Our struggles with mental illness or any kind of bodily suffering
need not weigh us down with guilt. As we pursue a new way of life,
we can experience freedom from the curse even while our bodies
suffer from the ills of a fallen creation. Theologian Joel Green writes
that 1 Peter takes an approach to resisting evil that fits well with
modern scientific ideas about how our behaviors and habits are
biologically and socially driven. In Green's own translation of the
verses, the apostle Peter writes that we are "no longer being shaped
by the desires that marked your former time of ignorance." Other
translations use the word "conform" rather than "shaped." But
"shaped" captures the fact that our desires, godly or sinful, are
molded by the world around us. Peter's letter "depicts sin as a power,
as 'worldly cravings that wage war against life.'" Because of this
power Peter emphasizes the importance of "the work of the Spirit
in hearing the good news and of a community set on following the
pattern of Christ and embodying the character of God."[8]

Peter's solution for this problem is to place us in an alternative
community under the power of the Spirit. Green writes: "The

Christian conception of human transformation [does not] allow us to think of the restoration of individuals, as it were, one at a time. . . . Persons are not saved in isolation from the world around them. Restoration to the likeness of God is the work of the Spirit within the community of God's people, the fellowship of Christ-followers set on maturation in Christ."[9]

Within this community we experience the reformation of our desires and hopes, the things we love and those we avoid. We are given a spiritual context in which to explore our experiences of suffering in light of the gospel. And we can pursue a new life that works to reduce our own suffering and that of others.

The cross frees us from guilt. The resurrection is our hope for new life in the midst of suffering. And the church is the site of our cultivation of a new way of life in which we pursue the good of ourselves while we care for others.

Made Perfect in Weakness

After Sally[10] broke out in hives, she finally skipped work to see a doctor. It had been an unusually stressful time at her office, not the best occasion to be ill at home. The doctor offered a treatment, but after hearing Sally describe being burdened at work, he recommended rest. Her body had reached its limit and was no longer able to deal with her stress-inducing environment. If she was to be healthy again, she needed respite. A real go-getter, Sally remarked, "I've just never been sick because of stress before." While she hadn't recognized the root causes of her suffering, her body was sending her clear signals. Her worry and anxiety were having physiological effects that she could no longer ignore.

We are a weakness-averse people. We pride ourselves on packed calendars, rigorous educations and strategic relationships. We see suffering and weakness as marks of inadequacy and failure. But, says J. I. Packer, we pay a price when we fail to come to terms with the depth of our brokenness. "We are all weak and inadequate, and need to face it," says Packer.

Sin, which disrupts all relationships, has disabled us all across the board. We need to be aware of our limitations and to let this awareness work in us humility and self-distrust, and a realization of our helplessness on our own. Thus we may learn our need to depend on Christ, our Savior and Lord, at every turn of the road, to practice that dependence as one of the constant habits of our heart, and hereby to discover what Paul discovered before us: "when I am weak, then I am strong" (2 Cor. 12:10).[11]

If we are to embrace our suffering not simply as the problem of pain but as a path toward deeper spiritual intimacy, we must be willing to accept our weakness.

Second Corinthians provides an excellent case study on accepting our limitations and embracing suffering. Throughout the book, Paul shows the church how suffering can be translated into strength as we rest in what Christ has done for us. "We do not want you to be uninformed, brothers and sisters, about the troubles we experienced," Paul writes. During their travels, he says, he and his companions feared for their lives. "But this happened that we might not rely on ourselves but on God, who raises the dead" (2 Cor 1:8-9).

Later in his letter, Paul affirms that suffering can result in a more intimate experience of faith. Often, he says, it is through our weaknesses that Christ works. We experience all kinds of hardships: "we are afflicted in every way, but not crushed; perplexed, but not driven to despair; persecuted, but not forsaken; struck down, but not destroyed." In fact, Paul writes, our experience of suffering is a "carrying in the body the death of Jesus, so that the life of Jesus may also be manifested in our bodies." And its purpose? A more intimate communion with and communication of Christ through our bodies—"so that the life of Jesus also may be manifested in our mortal flesh" (2 Cor 4:8-11 ESV).

Paul returns to the theme later in his letter, when he argues for his own qualifications as an apostle. But he turns boasting on its head when he says, "If I must boast, I will boast of the things that show my weakness" (2 Cor 11:30 ESV). Though he had been taken up into heaven and given visions, Paul cites his experience of chronic suffering as the place where his boasting could be most manifest.

To keep me from becoming conceited because of the surpassing greatness of the revelations, a thorn was given me in the flesh, a messenger of Satan to harass me, to keep me from becoming conceited. Three times I pleaded with the Lord about this, that it should leave me. But he said to me, "My grace is sufficient for you, for my power is made perfect in weakness." Therefore I will boast all the more gladly of my weaknesses, so that the power of Christ may rest upon me. For the sake of Christ, then, I am content with weaknesses, insults, hardships, persecutions, and calamities. For when I am weak, then I am strong. (2 Cor 12:7-10 ESV)

As he closes his letter, Paul once again relates his own weakness to that of the Suffering Servant. Even as Christ "was crucified in weakness, but lives by the power of God," so too is this power accessible for all believers who long for relief from suffering and for the day when the mortal is caught up in immortality (2 Cor 13:4 ESV). However we experience weakness, so did Christ. God subjected himself to this broken creation and to the cruelty and injustice of humanity. He experienced it fully, from ridicule and doubt to beatings and death.

As we recognize God's suffering in the person of Christ, our own pain finds its context, and we can experience a renewal of our relationship with God. In a remission following horrific cancer, the poet Christian Wiman found a companion in Jesus, whose sufferings allowed Wiman to feel as though someone understood his pain. Wiman's cancer had gotten into his bones, and as it spread and grew the expanding pressure on his bones was unbearable. When the pain of chemotherapy came, it killed the cancer in part, but his agony only increased. But Wiman, who had returned to faith in Jesus after decades away, found that Jesus removed the isolation produced by suffering.

> I am a Christian because of that moment on the cross when Jesus, drinking the very dregs of human bitterness, cries out, My God, my God, why hast thou forsaken me? . . . I am a Christian because I understand that moment of Christ's passion to have meaning in my own life, and what it means is that the absolutely solitary and singular nature of extreme human pain is an illusion. . . . I'm suggesting that Christ's suffering shatters the iron walls around individual human suffering, that Christ's compassion makes extreme human compassion—to the point of death, even—possible. Human love can reach right into death, then, but not if it is merely human love.[12]

Throughout the Bible, God works especially through human weakness, through our own broken bodies. Abraham was too old, Moses too cowardly, Gideon's army too insufficient, David too young and later too lustful, Elijah too alone, Jeremiah too persecuted. Yet within our weaknesses and through our sufferings God is present, he works, and he redeems.

Paul responded to suffering by looking for this final redemption. Uniquely, Paul expresses not a way out of suffering but a way *through* suffering to the fulfillment of all human longing, something far beyond what we can even imagine. He writes, "For while we are still in this tent, we groan, being burdened—not that we would be unclothed [not for escape], but that we would be further clothed, so that what is mortal may be swallowed up by life" (2 Cor 5:4 ESV). Packer sums up these verses saying,

> It is wonderful to know that somewhere in the process of transition out of the body into the next world, Christ himself will meet us, so that we may expect his face to be the first thing we become aware of in that new order of life into which we will have moved. Looking forward to this is the hope that will sustain us, as evidently it sustained Paul, while we grow older and our weaknesses, limitations, and thorns in the flesh increase.[13]

If we are to make peace with our suffering, we need not pretend it doesn't exist. Instead, as the grace of God makes us able, we can embrace our suffering and limitations as a path to deeper intimacy with God. As our bodies remind us of our frailty, we can draw closer to God, whose grace is sufficient and whose power is particularly evident in our weakness.

Weakness as Opportunity

In the past two years since Clarissa became sick, our family has felt deeply the limitations set by anxiety. And those limitations have changed the way we live. Our weekly schedule looks different, our expectations of our bodies have changed. Clarissa's suffering forced us to acknowledge her and our limitations in fundamental, physical ways. While that recognition has been deeply painful for her, Clarissa has found that failing to observe these limits involves high costs. But learning to live with limitations has also been a freeing process. In creating space for recovery, we have brought more health into our home. Her suffering has made us acutely aware of the weaknesses innate in the human body, and it has given us a deep longing to encourage those who walk a similar path.

When we seek to find Christ in our weakness, we don't simply look away to a future life without suffering. We look, as Paul did, for this broken mortality to be swallowed up by life. And one way we can do that is by responding to suffering with compassion. If prayer enhances our sense of compassion and our connection to other people, God has designed our bodies to respond to suffering. Often our response to others can alleviate our own suffering as we find encouragement in community.

In a study of 132 patients with multiple sclerosis (MS), researchers formed two groups, one of people who met weekly to learn coping skills and another of people who met monthly and received support from another person with multiple sclerosis. The goal was to see which group fared better, those learning coping skills or those hearing from another MS sufferer. The surprise finding was that neither group fared as well as did the five MS sufferers who had been trained to offer support. The study found that "giving support improved health more than receiving it." Those five MS sufferers felt a dramatic change in how they viewed themselves and life. Depression, self-confidence and self-esteem improved markedly. The main researcher said, "These people had undergone a spiritual transformation that gave them a refreshed view of who they were."[14] Caring for others brought healing for the caregivers.

Our nervous system is wired to find satisfaction—and discover our own well-being—by seeking the best for other people. "The emotions that promote the meaningful life are organized according to an interest in the welfare of others," says one researcher. "Compassion shifts the mind in ways that increase the likelihood of taking pleasure in the improved welfare of others."[15]

That is simply a scientific way of expressing the exhortation of Paul as he begins 2 Corinthians: "Blessed be the God and Father of our Lord Jesus Christ, the Father of mercies and God of all comfort, who comforts us in all our affliction, so that we may be able to comfort those who are in any affliction, with the comfort with which we ourselves are comforted by God. For as we share abundantly in Christ's sufferings, so through Christ we share abundantly in comfort too" (2 Cor 1:3-5).

Ed Dobson, a pastor and author, writes about how he has found more meaning caring for others with ALS, or Lou Gehrig's disease, since he himself was diagnosed with the degenerative disease. In his book *Seeing Through the Fog,* Dobson writes that the local ALS group asked him to visit others who had been recently diagnosed with ALS. So he does, every week.

> Over the years, I have talked with all sorts of people who have ALS. I talk with at least one individual every week. It might not seem as fancy as preaching to five thousand people, but it is powerful. When I look into their eyes, it's as if I am looking into their souls. Even when I'm talking on the phone, it's as if they are right there in the room with me. We are both broken. We both have a limited time on earth. We both know that dying is in our future. We both know that our muscles will

continue to decline. It's like we're on common ground. It's not a pastor up on the platform teaching truths to the congregation seated beneath him. It is one broken person talking to another broken person. And there is power in that.[16]

Oliver Sacks, the neurologist and author, says that "a disease is never a mere loss or excess—that there is always a reaction, on the part of the affected organism or individual, to restore, to replace, to compensate for and to preserve its identity, however strange the means may be."[17] It is in our reaction to suffering, how we respond to our pain, that God works in our weakness, comforting us as we comfort others, showing us his power in our weakness today. Suffering, real and terrible though it is, can uncover what is good and beautiful.

We need not enjoy our brokenness, but we must accept it. As we respond to suffering, and as the power of God is made perfect in our weakness, we participate today in the eventual and total repair of our world. We groan in our flesh now, desiring to be free from suffering. But as we embrace our suffering as a path to intimacy and reach beyond it to comfort others, we are enacting what God will do in the consummation of all things. We are bringing beauty out of pain, transforming our groans into glorious praise.

In a letter to his friend, St. Augustine complains about the distance separating them, and this distance prompts him to long for a heavenly kingdom. "I have no patience with that spurious 'strength of character' that puts up patiently with the absence of good things. Do we not all long for the future Jerusalem? . . . I cannot refrain from this longing: I would be inhuman if I could. Indeed, I derive some sweetness from my very lack of self-control; and, in this sweet yearning, I seek some small consolation."[18]

Though our present suffering may require patient endurance, our hearts are filled with a passionate yearning for the time when all that is broken will be fixed. Our suffering today is not the end of the story. As we seek Christ in our suffering and respond to others with Christ's comfort, we eagerly await the full realization of God's new creation, when "he will wipe every tear from their eyes. [And] there will be no more death or mourning or crying or pain" (Rev 21:4).

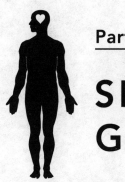

Part Two

SPIRITUAL GROWTH

PRACTICING
THE DISCIPLINES

FOLLOWING A PERIOD OF SUFFERING, it is common to hear someone say that despite the hardship they would go through it all again because it has made them a better person. The experience of suffering has forced a change in who they are that would not have been possible otherwise. Suffering shows that our experiences can fundamentally change who we are.

Unlike the normally involuntary shaping of suffering, the spiritual disciplines allows us to undertake experiences that can shape us in ways that we *choose*. Dallas Willard defines a discipline as "an activity within our power—something we can do—which brings us to a point where we can do what we at present cannot do by direct effort."[1]

"Christianity," says theologian Stanley Hauerwas, "is to have one's body shaped, one's habits determined, in such a manner that the worship of God is unavoidable."[2] But we often mold our bodies in ways to avoid worship, even though it's not what we want to do. We all face the problem that we are not the people we wish ourselves to be, and we also confront the disappointment that we have trouble choosing to become different than who we are. Whether we are striving to keep New Year's resolutions or forge a new path toward deep change, whether we want to exercise more and take better care of our bodies or to develop an intimate relationship with God, we have trouble controlling the reins that could direct our bodies down the paths we desire.

As Willard describes the process of spiritual formation, he says that God makes possible a new choice, but it is one that still requires effort. Though God doesn't force us into a new life, through the Spirit we are now free to choose differently. The good we wish to do, because of the new life within us, we can do. Even this freedom, says Willard, requires effort. Grace makes new life possible, but "it does not of itself restore the soul into the wholeness intended for it in its creation. . . . Rather, I must learn and accept the responsibility of moving with God in the transformation of my own personality. Intelligent and steady implementation of plans for change [is] required."[3]

These kinds of plans, Willard writes, usually fall under the category of spiritual disciplines. The disciplines shape our soul so that we become the kinds of people who naturally do the kinds of things that Jesus would want us to do. Richard Foster, a disciple of Willard, lists these disciplines in his book *Celebration of Discipline: The Path to Spiritual Growth*—practices like prayer, fasting, simplicity, service and confession

These disciplines work by shaping who we are through what we can do. The disciplines don't involve exercises in *not sinning.* Jesus tells us not to be anxious, for example, but the training offered by the spiritual disciplines is simplicity, the practice of seeking first the kingdom of God and discovering that "all these things" will be added to us. We do not discover relief from worries by trying to stave it off but by experiencing satisfaction in having fewer wants and needs in the pursuit of God's kingdom.

The disciplines change our being through our doing. That's because we shape our soul through our actions.

The Thinking Body

We can get a glimpse into how this works by understanding how our bodies shape our thinking. Well before we have conscious rational thoughts, our bodies are selecting and refining the pieces of information provided to our consciousness. The neuroscientist Antonio Damasio ran a fascinating experiment a couple decades ago that has become a famous example of how our bodies think and inform the thoughts in our minds.

Damasio shows that even our emotions result from the state of our bodies. In fact, when the brain is damaged in such a way that it cannot properly interpret the state of the body, people become unable to experience emotions such as fear and joy. For example, if a brain injury prevents your brain from sensing the high blood pressure, quick heartbeat and shortness of breath that accompany fear, it results in an inability to feel afraid.

What this shows is that the brain doesn't recognize a fearsome situation and begin a rapid heartbeat in response to feeling afraid. Instead, we become afraid when we experience the rapid heartbeat. Even if Damasio's patients could describe in detail how someone ought to feel in a situation, because of their brain injury they could not *experience* those emotions because they could not feel the state of their bodies. Crucially, this affected their rational thinking. The inability to interpret the state of the body, Damasio shows, disrupts a person's ability to reason. "Mind is probably not conceivable without some sort of *embodiment*," says Damasio.[4]

This is why the spiritual disciplines can change us. Active practices change our minds by shaping the habits of our bodies. Ideally, they make the worship of God unavoidable.

Damasio's experiment, retold in Malcolm Gladwell's book *Blink*,[5] is probably the most famous. He and his research team set up a card game and measured subjects' bodily responses as they learned to play. In the simple game, a player sits in front of four decks of cards. She can choose a card from any deck and, depending on the card, will either win or lose money. The decks have certain probabilities, however, with two of them offering big gains mixed intermittently with steady losses. Over time these losses are costly. The other decks offer smaller wins and losses, but over time these decks are winners. Damasio explains how typical gamblers react.

> What regular folks do in the experiment is interesting. They begin by sampling from all four decks, in search of patterns and clues. Then, more often than not, perhaps lured by the experience of high reward from turning cards in the A and B decks, they show an early preference for those decks. Gradually, however, within the first thirty moves, they switch the preference to decks C and D. In general, they stick to this strategy until the end.[6]

It makes sense that slowly, with experience, the players figure out how to win the game. But what the experiment also shows is how the gamblers came to know which decks would cost them money. Damasio performed the experiment again, this time with sensors on the subjects' skin that measured stress. We tend to sweat more when nervous, and Damasio found that his laboratory gamblers did just that whenever they chose a bad card. Their stress would shoot up with every loss.

But quickly, after turning over just ten cards, the gamblers' stress level would skyrocket *before* they overturned a card from the bad decks. This took only a handful of attempts, but Damasio could measure the stress on their skin before the players could consciously explain which decks were good or bad. As they played, they showed more and more stress associated with the bad decks. Consequently the gamblers began preferring good decks before they could consciously explain why.

Research widely accepts that all of our emotions are dependent on the feelings of our bodies. Our brains are constantly mapping the states of our bodies, and these states give rise to our feelings and emotions. Damasio has given empirical proof of the suggestion that psychologist William James offered a century ago:

> What kind of an emotion of fear would be left, if the feelings neither of quickened heart-beats nor of shallow breathing, neither of trembling lips nor of weakened limbs, neither of goose-flesh nor of visceral stirrings, were present, it is quite impossible to think. Can one fancy the state of rage and picture no ebullition of it in the chest, no flushing of the face, no dilatation of the nostrils, no clenching of the teeth, no impulse to vigorous action, but in their stead limp muscles, calm breathing, and a placid face?[7]

What Damasio's experiment shows is that our thoughts and desires arise from the activity of our bodies. We think of ourselves as having a command center, a central control for the decisions we make and the things we choose to do. But he and other researchers are changing that model. We ought not to think of ourselves as drivers of a car, with the ability to turn a wheel or press a pedal and expect a consistent, automatic result. Instead, in the image of one researcher, we are driving elephants. We have tools to control the elephant. We can poke and prod. We can encourage and inhibit. We can tame and train the elephant. But doing so requires discipline over time. Our conscious selves are not in full and immediate control, even if we aren't helpless in becoming who we seek to be.

Why the Spiritual Disciplines Work

We are accepted by God because of his love for us, not because of what we believe or our efforts to do the right things. But growth in love, patience, hope, goodness, faithfulness and all these traits of spiritual unity with Christ involves the disciplined actions of our bodies. As much as we intellectually assent to our faith, the actions of our bodies must be aligned to these thoughts for us to have any success in our spiritual growth. This alignment is what makes the spiritual disciplines so valuable. By pairing thought with action, the spiritual disciplines provide the routines necessary to train our bodies, and thus our minds as well, to follow after Jesus.

Neuroscience sheds light on how fasting and other spiritual disciplines work by training the subconscious mental processes that respond to the habits and desires of our bodies. Damasio's gambling subjects intuitively understood how to win the game before they could explain why the winning strategy worked. What this means for our spiritual lives is that we must develop our spiritual intuition through the activities we undertake. Before we consistently and consciously choose the things of God, we need to habitually feel and desire them.

For example, though there are many reasons to fast, studies suggest that at a very basic level this limited dose of self-control can increase a person's overall self-control. Fasting can train and shape the subconscious processes that regulate our desires. One study found that students who intentionally practiced good posture for a period of two weeks showed significant improvement afterward on measures of self-control.[8] In other words, practicing a low level of self-control gives us the ability to control ourselves in other ways.

The ability to control our relationship to food is, of course, one of the most difficult of the disciplines, but traditional fasting isn't starvation. Instead, on certain days of the year many Christians fast by eating something like a vegan diet. This kind of modest control over our intake, the kind that we can consciously choose, enables us to then control ourselves in other more significant ways. And when we fail—as we will—it teaches us a modest measure of humility.

As we consider how the brain directs the body, we must remember that there is no foreman of the brain barking out orders to subordinates. Every action we take changes our brains in a variety of ways. The connections between neurons strengthen or weaken, enabling or inhibiting our behaviors. "As far as we can tell," says neuroscientist David Eagleman, "all activity in the brain is driven by other activity in the brain, in a vastly complex, interconnected network." Since there is no command center in the brain, consciousness remains a mystery for scientists. When our good intentions go awry or our actions don't necessarily reflect our beliefs, we don't need to worry or mentally beat ourselves up. We are simply complex people with various competing impulses. Eagleman continues, "We don't find any spot in the brain that is not itself driven by other parts of the network. Instead, every part of the brain is densely interconnected with—and driven by—other brain parts."[9] An outcome of spiritual disciplines is to help these competing drives to instead work more consistently toward the same goals.

"Your most fundamental drives are stitched into the fabric of your neural circuitry," says Eagleman, "and they are inaccessible to you."[10] Or at least they are not *directly* accessible to you. There are limits to what we can accomplish by direct effort.

In his book *The Righteous Mind*, cognitive psychologist Jonathan Haidt says that our conscious minds are riders (not even drivers!) on the elephant of our subconscious mind and body. He lists six rules to help us understand this new way of thinking about the mind.

1. *Brains evaluate instantly and constantly.* Researchers have found that we immediately attach value judgments to the things we encounter, and those snap judgments are only later given rational justification. We feel first, then think.

2. *Social and political judgments are particularly intuitive.* Haidt and his colleagues have found that instant evaluations are especially true when it comes to other people and people groups. For example, liberals experience severe cognitive dissonance when they see words like "gun owners" and "compassion" put together. Even when given no context for these words, their brains create a context in which to interpret them. The same occurs for conservatives when they see words like "pro-choice" and "love."

3. *Our bodies guide our judgments.* Whether subjects washed their hands or smelled foul odors during questions, all affected their responses. People with clean hands, for example, were more likely to feel disgust toward immoral ideas. Your moral judgments are not merely the reasoned consequence of your biblical worldview.

4. *Psychopaths reason but don't feel.* Lacking these instinctive feelings is the definition of a psychopath, whose reasoning is almost perfectly intact. He or she simply has no feelings. G. K. Chesterton was exactly right: "The madman is not the man who has lost his reason. He is the man who has lost everything except his reason."[11]

5. *Babies feel but don't reason.* Researchers have found that our brains work this way from the very start, and that our reasoning only develops later. It seems as though a baby's social world is similar. "By six months of age, infants are watching how people behave toward *other people,* and they are developing a preference for those who are nice rather than those who are mean." Our intuitions are largely inborn.

6. *Affective reactions are in the right place at the right time in the brain.* So far, all the research has suggested that our emotional processing is primary; cognitive thinking and rationalization come later. When researchers looked at brain scans as people made moral judgments, they found exactly what they should have. The areas of the brain making moral choices are the emotional areas, not the rational ones.[12]

These rules suggest the degree to which our conscious minds are not in charge of our thoughts and desires. Our instinctive feelings and emotions matter far more than rational ideas or worldviews. This isn't to say that our frontal lobes, which perform our cognitive processing, are irrelevant. We can change our instincts. We can think through an emotional reaction and, with time and effort, reverse course. Experiences with other people can help us do the same. If we are to have any success in cultivating spiritual disciplines, we must be willing to hold in tension the reality that we are able to direct our course and yet we are also subject to our own frailty.

David Brooks writes in *The Social Animal,* "The key to a well-lived life is to have trained the emotions to send the right signals and to be sensitive to their subtle calls."[13] We train our emotions, the feelings of our subconscious that arise to awareness, by taking on new behaviors. Timothy Wilson, professor of psychology at the University of Virginia, says this is how we train those "fundamental drives stitched into the fabric of our neural circuitry. . . . The more frequently people perform a behavior, the more habitual and automatic it becomes, requiring little effort or conscious attention. One of the most enduring lessons of social psychology is that behavior change often precedes changes in attitude and feelings."[14]

This is how the spiritual disciplines work, shaping the kinds of instinctive reactions we are likely to have from the bottom up. The disciplines allow us to instinctively pursue God rather than relying on the weaker executive control. Rather than needing to choose the things of God, we become the kinds of people who desire them and pursue them because that is what we love.

We often talk about the disciplines as useful reminders. Fasting helps us pray because our hunger reminds us of our dependence on God. But prayer, meditation on Scripture and all other spiritual disciplines are not simply reminders like strings tied to our fingers. Instead, they shape our emotions. The disciplines teach and enable us to live by deeper truths and in accord with a deeper reality than the basic cravings of our bodies.

Do First, Then Feel

Sheldon Mann, a health care chaplain in Southern California, illustrates how the disciplines—not simply changed belief—can change someone's life. Sheldon grew up in a harsh environment and was subjected to sexual, physical and emotional abuse. His parents divorced when he was seven, and Sheldon said goodbye to his dad and older brother. In San Francisco's East Bay, a tough school and community environment, combined with Sheldon's home, made living insufferable. "I was in a very bad area," he says, "very violent."

At thirteen years old, Sheldon was playing drums in a band, drinking alcohol and doing drugs.

His life changed after two girls invited him to play drums with a church youth choir. "I said they were crazy," he says, but he took them up on the offer. What he saw was "mesmerizing." The folks at church had something about them that Sheldon just couldn't understand. "Whatever they had I wanted," he says. "Six months later I heard about grace, sin and Christ. I became a believer."

Sheldon went to a Christian college, he got married, and he moved to Texas, where he and his wife started their family. Eventually they had three children. But while Sheldon knew that his sins had been forgiven by the grace of Christ, his growing-up years had deeply scarred him. Even regular churchgoing and his Christian college studies did not heal those scars.

"I had a huge anger issue," Sheldon says, "because I grew up the way I did." These personal flaws would contribute to ending his marriage. "That is probably one of the huge character flaws that I've had," he says. Formerly he thought, *When someone comes at you, you put up a protective barrier, never appear vulnerable, and let others know there is a real danger as quickly as possible.* It took years of spiritual practice for Sheldon to see the unhealthiness of those instincts. He wasn't able to see how his anger and lack of control were a problem when it mattered, when his marriage depended on it.

Sheldon describes his divorce as "a tough, tough thing. I wouldn't wish that on my worst enemy," he says. "I was really mad at God. Though he wouldn't let me turn my back on him, he let me crash and burn." He went back to smoking and drinking; he dated other women. "I lost everything," Sheldon says; "I was empty."

Looking back, Sheldon compares himself to the prodigal son. It was only after he had left God and squandered all that he had that Sheldon thought it might have been better in his "father's house." After eight years, he says, his the emptiness of his lifestyle compelled him to return to Jesus Christ.

Sheldon left his career at United Parcel Service and his home in Texas and went to work for his brother in Southern California. After eight months he began to hear God calling him back to ministry. "This was unexpected, and I felt that I was having some kind of emotional break. This kept happening every day for the next three weeks, and at one point I told God that he was out of his mind for choosing me." Finally, one day while arguing with God, Sheldon said, "I am not the guy! I am selfish, I have hurt and used others; I do not see how I can be of any good use for your kingdom."

But Sheldon still felt God's call as well as a sense that God would take care of all of his own character flaws. Sheldon's job was to follow Jesus. "I took him at his word and began to clean up all the questionable areas of my life." After months of prayer, Sheldon enrolled at Talbot School of Theology at Biola University in Los Angeles. He was then offered an unusual opportunity, one in which God would make good on his promise to take care of Sheldon's personal problems. A federal official needed someone to watch his desert property. The agent would unwind there after dealing with high-profile, dangerous cases, but the property needed looking after between those infrequent visits. Sheldon accepted the assignment.

In that remote location, Sheldon took up residence in a small cabin with electricity, running water and propane hooked to a gas stove. It stood in the middle of the San Diego Mountain Desert. There was no phone or television. "The hardest thing at first was the intense loneliness. I've never been any place that quiet," he says. For three weeks it was nearly unbearable. A few times a week each semester he would commute two hours to get to class, but outside of those excursions, his only companion was God. "You start having a conversation with God out there," he says. "It becomes more of a narrative. It's a constant conversation."

Sheldon decided to make the most of the opportunity and use his two years at that cabin as a place for quiet and contemplation, he says, "a place for research and study, with no one and nothing to take away my attention and focus."

It was there that Sheldon confronted his inner anger. "As I became more aware of sin and areas of my life that I'd buried or that I had become accustomed to that I thought were okay, God brought my attention to the things I had to work out." Sheldon's confrontation with his sinful self sent him into a deep depression that lasted a month. "I went into mourning for my past, my children, the wrongs I had done. There was a deep, deep pain, intense weeping."

Sheldon realized that his sin went even deeper than anger. He harbored a selfish sense of entitlement. "I was very self-absorbed," he says. "I was going to take what I wanted." This painful recognition, he believes, could only have been born of the intense prayer and the work of the Holy Spirit he experienced in that lonely desert place.

Finally, he says, "I understood God through Christ forgave me."

Out in the desert, his sense of God deepened, and he grew more attuned to the spiritual, unseen aspects of existence. "It was the most worshipful experience of my life," he says. After those two years of solitude and silence, he had a communion with God that he didn't want to lose. "I really enjoy the relationship when you can interact with the Lord and walk with him. There is nothing that appeals to me more than that relationship. Nothing else holds me."

Today at times the old anger will rise up, usually because of a perceived slight or offense. "I still get my ears up," Sheldon says. "But I don't take it personally anymore. I wonder what's hurting that person. I've learned to release that through prayer and the Spirit working through it."

Sheldon attributes his change to his discipline of prayer and solitude, but, interestingly, not to his seminary studies, even though he graduated with two master's degrees, in the philosophy of religion and in theology. Certainly the content of his classes gave him much to feast upon, but it was only in the desert—a place that required spiritual discipline—that Sheldon was able to trust Jesus Christ to make the changes that would shape his spiritual life and growth as a believer.

My Spiritual Cycle

Most of us are not able to hunker down in the desert to focus on spiritual growth. More often our spiritual development comes in the midst of our workaday world, sandwiched between chauffeuring the kids to soccer practice and preparing for a board meeting. Still, here in the mundane routines of our day, the spiritual disciplines can quietly begin to reshape our minds as they introduce new patterns into our behavior.

A number of years ago, during an hour-long commute, I started listening to the Bible. I'd run out of audiobooks and picked up a few Bible CDs. After a few car rides full of Scripture, my commute turned into church. Hearing the Bible read for an hour can do that.

During that period of prayer and Scripture listening, I finally understood the power of the spiritual disciplines. My life with God was no longer tossed by the winds of my enthusiasm; I now set my own course. Each morning and each evening, my routine dictated my spiritual development. It was incredibly powerful.

Over time, I became more attuned to my spiritual health. I became more sensitive to my responses to others, more ready to acknowledge when I had reacted in frustration or anger to something at work or at home. In the same way that eating healthily gives me a taste for healthful foods, the spiritual disciplines gave me a craving for more. Now when my life went out of alignment, I could feel it—and do something about it. I could return to the practices that had fed my soul and prompted me toward Christlikeness.

In ways that are almost imperceptible at first to our conscious minds, the spiritual disciplines begin to grow us to be more like Christ. We can use fasting, meditation, prayer or another rhythm to guide this development, and we must be patient. It may take years, as it did for Sheldon, to see the fruits of our commitment. But we can be assured that our brains are reforming as our practices help to mold us more into the image of Jesus. Changing who we are requires more than church services and good theology. To change our being, to make us spiritually sensitive beings, we need to take up the practices that make us the kinds of people who desire to live out a love for God and our neighbors.

WORSHIP

Engaging the Senses

WHY DOES A PERSON GO TO CHURCH? As someone who was helping to plant a church, I often asked myself this question. What brings people in, and what makes them stay? The success of our little church plant would depend on our finding those answers. Most evangelical church services consist of preaching and music, but if I could fill my iPod with sermons from the world's best preachers and worship music from Christian musicians, why show up on a Sunday morning? If church's main elements were available to me on my sofa, why not stay at home in my pajamas?

It appears that even as early as the book of Hebrews, the church was struggling against those questions. Saints were charged to not give up "meeting together, as some are in the habit of doing" (Heb 10:25). Others had to be reminded that the purpose of gathering wasn't to stuff their bellies with food (1 Cor 11:20-22). They, like we, brought their expectations to church. For those of us who seek to obey the words of Scripture, participating in regular worship, the sacraments and the faith community is our duty as believers. There is a neurological reason that these habits are good for us as well.

Worship allows us to experience our belief in union with fellow believers, making the content of our belief more meaningful and life changing. In the words of a pair of researchers, through worship or ritual, belief "becomes an experienced fact."[1] This experience of theology is made powerful by the community in which we worship and the rich, complex way that our brains process experiences.

Philosopher James K. A. Smith argues that Christians have focused too heavily on educating our minds to the neglect of training our hearts. We are people, he says, "whose orientation to the world is shaped from the body up more than from the head down. Liturgies aim our love to different ends precisely by training our hearts through our bodies."[2] At its most powerful, worship balances the mind and the body in a way that we can experience union with God, transforming our nature.

Worship can lead us into experiences of God, whether sublime or profound, that shape our hearts. Worship can give us an experience of God himself, in unity with fellow worshipers, and in a theologically rich, multisensory environment full of meaning. It forms our desires and shapes our emotions, making us more like Christ, uniting heaven and earth, creation and Creator. But it's not until we get off the sofa and into the pew that we are able to experience these things.

Converted by Worship

One thousand years ago when the Russians converted to Christianity, they were as unlikely to become Christian as any "unchurched" skeptic might be today. In the tenth century, after the Russians—formerly a tribe of Vikings—settled into kingdom building, they realized they were better off participating in the economic order rather than stealing from it. Prince Vladimir determined that the Viking religion was a thing of the past, so he sent emissaries to nearby tribes to learn of their faith. The Bulgars' mosque was disappointing. "There is no happiness among them, but instead only sorrow and a dreadful stench." German Catholic worship was dull. The emissaries also passed on the Judaism to which the Khazars of central Asia had converted. Attempts to Christianize the Russians had failed in the past. Missionaries had baptized Vladimir's grandmother. The missionary brothers Cyril and Methodius had provided an alphabet (the Cyrillic alphabet now in use) for the Slavic languages and translated the Bible into it, but it hadn't yet had much effect on the Russians. Trade with the Byzantines led to a number of individual conversions, but Christianity remained a minority among the Rus. The Russians had a history of violently opposing the faith. The Vikings had been sacking churches, murdering priests and enslaving Christians for three hundred years. Nevertheless, following a single visit to a church in Constantinople, a delegation returned to Russia convinced that the kingdom needed to convert.

In 988, when Vladimir's delegation of transplanted Vikings visited, the leaders of the church in Constantinople put the full glories of Byzantine worship on display for their Russian visitors. The delegation was brought to the Hagia Sophia, the crown jewel of Byzantine worship, built by Emperor Justinian in the sixth century. Supported by forty arched windows that allowed the sun to stream in, the dome appeared to be "suspended from heaven by a golden chain"[3] high above the worshipers. Other windows focused sunshine like a galaxy of stars across the walls and ceiling. Light would have sparkled off the gold mosaics, which covered the interior space and provided illustration for the Scripture readings that filled the worship services. Every corner of the church provided an opportunity for devotion, with objects of meditation tucked into every crevice. The icons, the intricate artistic detail, candles and incense all spoke to the ardent devotion of the Christians who worshiped there. And there were thousands. The worship space was expansive, and worship was orchestrated by more than five hundred people in specific serving roles.[4]

When the Russian delegation arrived, they were overawed. "The Greeks led us to the edifices where they worship their God," they reported back to Vladimir, "and we knew not whether we were in heaven or on earth. For surely there is no such splendor or beauty anywhere on earth. We cannot describe it to you: Only this we know, that God dwells there among humans, and that their service surpasses the worship of all other places. For we cannot forget that beauty."[5]

The Orthodox Church provides a unique perspective on worship that many of us as post-Reformation Christians have lost. Instead of being a useful multipurpose building, the Orthodox church structure continues to be primarily a worship space. The emphasis on beauty is informed by theology. "When Orthodox believers entered into such a church, they were presented with a structure that revealed neither a remote God nor a mere image. Rather, Patriarch Photius [of ninth-century Constantinople] insisted, such a structure was anchored in 'truth and reality' and revealed 'grace and Spirit.'"[6] The "smells and bells" are intended to provide an experience of belief, feeding all the senses. The richer and more complex the experience, neurologically the more powerfully worshipers experience the meaning and the theology attached to it.

By offering more than biblical tips for living, Byzantine worship, like Orthodox worship today, cultivated a strong Christian identity and a lifestyle of devotion among its followers. "The Church is heaven on earth," said the eighth-century Patriarch Germanus I.[7] While the church building used stone and painting to symbolically unite heaven and earth, the liturgy guided worshipers into a sense of union with God. "The tradition has not been content simply to proclaim Christ in words alone but has developed a ritual that is full of visual splendor, with grand gestures meant to be seen and understood by all."[8]

The Orthodox want their worship to bring believers into a close experience of Christ so that through it they become more holy. The Orthodox seek *theosis* or deification, in which Christians take on the nature of Christ. For these believers, becoming Christlike isn't merely about doing what Jesus would do but about becoming who Jesus was. We can partake of the divine nature, as Peter put it (2 Pet 1:4), so that our nature itself becomes more holy. "As Archbishop Symeon of Thessalonika says, the purpose of liturgy is the same as the incarnation, namely, that believers 'become partakers of God . . . according to grace.'" Worship, therefore, "is an encounter that is at once personal and corporate, brought about by both a direct experience and a remembrance of God's salvific work."[9]

Orthodox worship seeks holiness by placing demands on its members. Worshipers fast before Communion, and they stand most of the service. The service I visited seemed to be largely made up of prayers sung back and forth between the congregation and the priests. Newcomers will spend a lot of time trying to follow and understand all that is happening, but it is a service that can dig itself deep into your soul.

The unique multisensory experience of worship in an Orthodox church serves as a powerful example as we explore how worship affects our bodies and our relationships with God and others. If we previously felt bound to the two-part model of worship—preaching and music—both the Orthodox experience and science invite us to expand our definitions of what worship looks like and explore new ways of fostering deep devotion as we participate in corporate worship.

Addicted to Worship

Ancient Orthodox worship isn't the only way that Christians have sought to make their praise reflect the connection between heaven and earth. Modern megachurch worship can have a similar effect on participants. Researchers at the University of Washington investigated twelve megachurches and conducted numerous interviews with attendees. They found that worship in these churches builds on oxytocin to produce a feeling of connectedness, taking social connection even further by integrating a sense of the divine.

To understand worship, the researchers compared it to another common measure of social euphoria, emotional energy. Social euphoria is present to some extent in any large gathering—a high school pep rally, a holiday parade or a Super Bowl party. The researchers defined social euphoria as "a bodily phenomenon . . . a feeling of confidence, courage to take action, boldness in taking initiative. It is a morally suffused energy; it makes the individual feel not only good, but exalted, with the sense of doing what is most important and most valuable."[10]

While there are many social gatherings that can produce emotional energy, such as a sporting event, a corporate conference or a political rally, the researchers added another component to their study to reflect the sense of spiritual connection that worshipers find in church. In their interviews with worshipers, the researchers found that they "discussed their experiences as being in contact with the divine, generally causing them to grow spiritually. For example, individuals described being in 'God's presence,' 'falling in love with Jesus,' being 'transformed,' and feeling that 'the Holy Spirit was here.'"[11]

Neurologically speaking, church worshipers' brains release the oxytocin that causes us to feel good about being with other people.

"When oxytocin levels rise, defensive postures decrease, levels of trust increase."[12] It is a highly addictive substance, which is a biological explanation for why, for many people, worship feels so necessary at least weekly. Oxytocin is also used to help addicts withdraw from heroin, which is why nearly every article written about the University of Washington study said that God is like a drug.

The emotional component of worship aids the instruction provided in the sermon. Our brains don't only think rationally, but cognition comes wedded to our guts, with our emotions. When we are emotionally tied to the worship service, we are primed to hear, believe and apply the Scripture that is taught.

The University of Washington researchers found that megachurch members felt connected to the teaching as well as the worship songs. Many members weren't initially attracted by the pastor's sermons. One interview subject said, "His message didn't bring [us] in. It was the attitude of the entire congregation," who welcomed them and exuded joy in worship. Yet eventually people came to depend on the teaching offered. "I don't want to miss the message," said one person, perhaps a little desperately; "I don't know if I'm going to get the message that God intends for me to get if I go someplace else." Continued attendance further increased the sense of need. "I just need to get it in," one person said; "it feels tangible, I was thirsting for God."

This social component gives worship a powerful appeal. It becomes more than a great concert, an exciting rally or an epic sporting event. Worship can connect worshipers to one another while each is experiencing the presence of God. And unlike at a concert, worshipers leave a church service with a sense of ultimate meaning. This unique combination of factors allows us to experience a strong connection to God that is unavailable in any other way. It may be a driving factor behind megachurch worship success. However, there is more to worship than connecting people to one another and to God at the same time.

Multisensory Worship

While experiencing God with other people is a powerful component of worship, a church service can do even more to lead us toward God, making use of the complex ways our brains process experiences. Many Christians have scrubbed their churches of the sights and smells of ancient liturgical rites, replacing them with generic mood-enhancing lighting or images. Nevertheless, those old traditions developed for a reason, and there is a neurological cost when worshipers look and act more like an audience, seated in chairs watching performances on stage, than like active participants in the service.

No matter what churches have done to their adult service, there is often one place where movement, pictures, chanting and similar practices have remained. Visit any children's Sunday school or worship room, and your senses are likely to be flooded. With children, we often need to integrate the senses in worship, since they simply won't sit still for an extended lesson. We sing songs that teach—rather than only songs that express feelings—and we add motions that help children remember the words. We teach Bible verses and use color charts to help children remember them and other theological concepts.

We have added these richer dimensions to our children's worship because we have learned they are effective in helping children learn. Indeed, research into how our brains learn and remember shows us why this is so. It isn't because they are children that these methods work; it's because they are human, though children may be more obviously receptive to a more experiential service. If we found ways to add some of these elements to our contemporary forms of worship, we would likely find that adults learn better this way as well. We might find that our worship experience becomes richer and enhances worshipers' opportunity to leave a service having not only learned about God but been changed by God.

When we consider how we can shape worship to allow participants the most benefit, we must look at how our brains store information. Contrary to popular belief, our brains do not record information like a tape player or a computer. This information is not stored somewhere in a file that we can access when we need the content. That may be how we *experience* our memories, playing them back from start to finish as if they were recorded on a videotape. But memory is more complex.

John Medina is a developmental molecular biologist at the University of Washington, where he studies how the brain handles information. He uses an entirely different metaphor for how our brains store information: a blender with the lid off.

When information enters our brains, it is sliced to shreds and then stored in various places inside our head. Medina writes, "The information is fragmented and redistributed the instant the information is encountered. If you look at a complex picture, for example, your brain immediately extracts the diagonal lines from the vertical lines and stores them in separate areas. Same with color. If the picture is moving, the fact of its motion will be extracted and stored in a place separate than if the picture were static."[13]

Before books were widespread, people had to memorize much more information than we would imagine is possible today, and they intuitively used this method. They handled this task by creating "memory palaces" in which different buildings and different rooms held different kinds of information. In a sense, this method made information more complex. You not only had to remember what you were trying to remember but also the mental palace you constructed and the details of the "room" in which the information was stored. However, by making the information more complex, this method actually utilized our brain's neurological method of storing memory.

Medina tells the story of a woman whose stroke made her unable to use written vowels, a phenomenon that told researchers that vowels are recognized by a different part of the brain from consonants. But it gets more complicated. If asked to write a sentence, the woman would include spaces where the vowels were supposed to be, telling researchers that even the placement of vowels in words was stored in yet another place.

When our brains present stored information to us, it seems like a unified whole. So it feels counterintuitive that all the bits and pieces of an experience are splattered across our brains. Even more surprising is that the more complex the information—the more bits and pieces to splatter throughout the brain—the easier it is for us to remember the information. Our experiences seem to be richer the more sights, sounds, smells and especially meaning that the experience involves. The richer the experience, the more powerful the memory and the easier it will be for us to remember. Since memory works by changing the physical structure of our brain, strengthening and loosening ties between neurons, experientially richer worship changes us more powerfully.

Think of it like this. If I were to ask you to remember the numbers 7, 12 and 40 then repeat them to me in a month, you might or might not be able to do it. But your likelihood of doing so would be dramatically increased if I reminded you of three facts: (1) It was on the seventh day that God rested. (2) Twelve is the number of the tribes of Israel and Jesus' disciples. (3) And forty is the number of years Israel spent in the wilderness, the number of days Jesus spent fasting before being tempted by the devil, and the number of days Jesus spent with his disciples after the resurrection. It might even help if I suggested that to help remember 7 you could think of the color green, to remind you of creation. You could think of brown for the number 12, to remind you that the disciples wore sandals. And you might think of yellow for the number 40, to remind you of the hot sun of the Sinai wilderness.

The complexity of meaning matters. Even further, the complexity of experience enhances our memories.

Medina writes that researchers know that words and pictures presented alongside each other make learning far more powerful. That's why PowerPoint presentations—when done well—can be effective. Because of the way our brains slice and dice the information we receive, adding related details in a different medium can make memory and learning easier. PowerPoint with words competes with the speaker's words, but PowerPoint with pictures adds richness.

Interestingly, adding smell to the equation can then double memory capacity. Because of the unique way that smell is processed in the brain, bypassing a central authority and passing its information directly to other parts of the brain, adding odor to information can make test subjects twice as likely to remember that information. Perhaps that's why incense is so often added to religious ceremonies. When we add complexity to the smell—by giving the incense meaning in which it is the fragrance of our worship rising to God—then the incense becomes even more powerful as an aid to worship.

Children need "motions" to help them listen. When worshipers stand, kneel, raise their hands, cross themselves or bow their heads, they are adding neurological richness to their experience. Their experience becomes more powerful, more likely to promote change.

All of these things—sights, smells, sounds—are not simply the stuff of children's Sunday school but integral ways in which we can experience God. If we are to learn how to worship with our whole selves, we must consider expanding the ways we worship to embrace how our brains engage our hearts. We may consider ancient liturgical traditions, or we may explore entirely new ways of engaging the senses. Whatever ways we choose, we will be enriching our worship as we connect to others and connect to God.

Training Our Bodies

A few years ago I attended two very different church services in the space of eight days, both of them employing the elements covered in this chapter. First, I worshiped in Rwanda at a nondenominational Pentecostal church. PowerPoint slides offered a mix of Bible texts and images of nature, and the singing was so enthusiastic that I felt swept up in it, creating a powerful social experience of a group united in worship. The preaching, at least an hour of it, began slow and calm, but it wasn't long before the preacher was in the middle of congregation prophesying and anointing people with oil. Members stood in praise while the preacher shouted into his microphone. There were no spectators here. Men, women, teenagers and the elderly—all were drawn into this powerful bodily experience of the presence of God.

A week later, back in the States, I attended the traditional Anglican service of my home church. I stood, knelt, sang and recited prayers throughout the service. The Bible, an illuminated edition by the artist Makoto Fujimura, was carried, lifted high, to the center of the congregation for the Gospel reading. The worship space was visually rich, filled with brightly decorated fabrics and handcrafted Eucharistic vessels. Worshipers sang with enthusiasm, accompanied by the priest on an acoustic guitar. Spontaneous as well as written prayers were offered, and worshipers had occasion to meet each other's eyes in welcome during the passing of the peace.

There may have been few visible similarities between these congregations half a world away from one another. But they share the same passionate pursuit of God, with worship that draws the congregation into deep connection with God and others. There is no prescribed method for how worship must work. Any church tradition can use these neurological principles of combining social elation, complex, rich learning experiences and connection with God to powerfully shape the hearts of worshipers.

Perhaps for too long we have emphasized information over experience. Or maybe we have prized experience so highly that theology gets short shrift. But when we understand how our bodies and our brains experience God in worship, we can work to shape our churches into places that can more personally and powerfully change lives. Worship makes us more Christlike by taking the content of our belief—theological abstractions—and allowing us to feel it alongside other believers. Beliefs become alive in us when worship combines the emotions of a social experience with a multisensory package of meaning. Then church can not only instruct our minds but change the orientation of our lives.

9

ACTS OF SERVICE

As an adult, my friend Jeff struggled with having been raised as a Christian. He wandered from the faith but couldn't fully escape it. He once told me, "I grew up in the church. It's in me. I don't have a choice here. I either find my way back to God or I struggle with the fact that I can't."

The tether pulling Jeff back to the faith—and troubling his life away from church—wasn't simply that he had grown up attending services, going to Christian camp in the summer and reading the Bible. Additionally, memories of his parents' acts of service in their church community nagged at him; their genuine love for others had been so apparent, it was hard to argue against a faith that called its followers to behave like that.

Throughout his life, Jeff's family had showed compassion to neighbors in need and opened their home to others. Long after Jeff started a family of his own and moved out of state, his parents continued to rearrange their lives in order to care for other people. Often they would adopt a person in need—a neighbor who was getting over some family trouble or a college student who had to take a semester off in order to earn money for next year's tuition. Neighbors would drop in regularly for meals or to request a cup of flour, borrow a toilet plunger or do laundry. Jeff's family's front door seemed to be a revolving one, always turning open for someone in need.

Jeff's family regularly demonstrated compassion, an action that may have been the greatest factor in his adult faith. Studies show that one of the most important influences on faith is routine acts of compassion. As an adult, Jeff might have had little trouble walking away from church attendance, but seeing his parents' faith in action, demonstrated by regular acts of service to others, caused Christianity to beckon to him even amidst his doubts.

Faith with Works

Scripture commands us to care for others, but this exhortation is far more than an abstract instruction. Our bodies are designed to recognize when someone needs our care and to respond. In fact, we become our best selves when we are focused on the needs of other people.

After studying the faith practices of a number of Christian families, Diana Garland was struck by the fact that aside from attending worship together, many families considered community service to be the most important thing they did as an expression of their faith. Garland, dean of the Baylor University school of social work, decided to follow up her discovery with another study. She surveyed 7,300 people in thirty-five congregations, seeking to "learn about the connection these Christians made between their life of faith and their involvement in community service." Her findings "changed how we think about church and how we think about being faithful as Christians."[1]

By comparing those who engage in voluntary community service with those who don't, Garland found that people who volunteer also pray and read the Bible more often. Not only that, but she found that service "had a more profound relationship with the faith of these ordinary Christians than any other faith activity, including attending congregational worship." Many might assume that great preaching or music attracts people to a particular church. But it appears that acts of service speak loudest when drawing those outside of the church and keeping followers in the faith.[2]

For teens as well, Garland found that service was the most important factor in developing their faith, more essential than Sunday school, youth worship or Bible study. Yet students weren't getting the opportunities to serve that they wanted. A Gallup survey found that while 60 percent of teens said they would like to be involved in church-based service projects, only 20 percent actually were.[3] But anecdotally, a friend confirmed Garland's results for me. In a church he attended, youth leaders offered no youth programming— no lock-ins, no outings, no special classes. Instead they simply emphasized service, and as a result the church couldn't keep young people away.

Garland hypothesizes that service may be so essential to young people's faith because in our world where careers don't begin until the early twenties, teens and young adults have few opportunities to do meaningful activities that contribute to the well-being of others. In a world where careers so define people's identity, children and young people flounder without defined roles and struggle to find meaningful service opportunities until their third decade in life. When our faith instruction so often emphasizes good behavior, acts of service can offer young people a less rule-based approach to faith that promotes their dedication and enthusiasm.

The proof of the link between faith and service can be seen by looking at churches and Christian families, and also by looking at people who volunteer. In their study of religion in America, Harvard sociologist Robert Putnam and Notre Dame political scientist David Campbell found that religious Americans were more likely to volunteer their time and donate their money than were non-religious Americans. Not only did churchgoers give more of their time and money overall, but they also gave more to *secular* causes than did secular Americans. In fact, while they did find some secular Americans who gave money to solely secular causes, for the most part American giving is by people who attend religious services and give to both religious and secular causes.

Putnam and Campbell report, "The most secular fifth of our sample reported an average of about $1,000 in total annual household charitable contributions, as compared to more than $3,000 for the most religious fifth. Measuring charitable giving as a fraction of annual income, the average person in the most religious fifth of Americans is more than four times as generous as his or her counterpart in the least religious fifth, roughly 7 percent vs. roughly 1.5 percent."[4] Compared to secular Americans, regular churchgoers volunteered an extra 10.5 hours per month for religious causes *and* an additional 6.4 hours per month for secular causes.[5] Looking at the kinds of activities that the faithful spend their time giving to, it is service to the poor, the elderly and young people where religious volunteers really stand out.

Whether we look at acts of service from inside the church, where it is linked to greater faith, or from the religious and secular organizations that benefit from the gifts of time and money offered largely by religious Americans, it is clear that service and faith are closely related. This research suggests that it wasn't just coincidence that during my training at a secular hospice organization near Chicago, every other volunteer attended church.

Hardwired for Compassion

People often are surprised to hear that I spent three years as a hospice volunteer. Those who haven't experienced hospice usually appear amazed. "Wow, it takes a special kind of person to be able to do that. You must really be passionate about it," they say. I've met foster parents who hear the same kinds of expressions from others. There are complexities to spending time with the dying or opening your home to a child who is not your own, but it's certainly not dependent upon superhuman levels of compassion.

I have learned to respond by simply saying that the only thing a person needs is the willingness to show up. Like foster parenting, hospice work is not highly specialized. It requires no special skills. Hospice volunteer coordinators might try to match people's interests—card players with other card players, for example—but otherwise there is little attempt after the initial training to find or develop a volunteer's skills. All that is required is the faithfulness to show up for the job.

As a hospice volunteer, I provided weekly companionship, often to patients who were very much alone. My faithful arrival each week allowed the patients I visited to feel the dignity that comes from knowing people still cared about them.

I'll admit, it wasn't easy. For example, I could never have a real conversation with my Alzheimer's patient. I remember going up the elevator to Edward's floor and thinking up topics I might chat about. I would ask him questions, and he would blather unintelligible sentences in reply. After a year I thought that perhaps he had begun to recognize me, but even that was hard to discern. Volunteering didn't give me goose bumps of excitement. I didn't feel a great sense of accomplishment for the work I did. In fact, often I wondered if my presence there was really making a difference, though research told me that it was. Many weeks I arrived simply because I had agreed to do so.

In my three years, two significant exceptions to this stand out. My first moment of joy in the year I visited Edward was when I met his wife. He was living in a government-run convalescent center, so I could never find out any personal information about his family or his past. However, on one occasion I ran into his wife in the hallway. When she realized who I was and why I was there, joy spread across her face. Someone had been visiting her husband every week. Seeing her delight and receiving her thanks gave me a rush of happiness. I was suddenly so glad to be visiting this man and eager to return the next week.

The second and final time I felt good about visiting him came, surprisingly, when I heard he had died. I fought back tears when I received the call. I had no idea how much this man, whose mind had long ago been destroyed, had come to mean to me. I knew very little about him, but knowing that I had done my part to care for him had suddenly, upon learning of his death, come to mean a great deal. Deeply saddened to hear of his death, I also sensed the incredible honor of having visited him and offered companionship during the last year of his life.

No one needs to spend months visiting an Alzheimer's patient to experience the benefits of compassionate service. Our everyday acts of kindness toward others, giving to good causes and generosity of time will consistently provide the joy that comes from helping out. When scientists put their students into labs and have them give each other trivial financial gifts, almost universally the students receive surges of joy that can actually be measured in brain chemicals.

We are hardwired for compassion, to tangibly express our love for our neighbors, and we are designed to *want* to do this because it makes us feel so incredibly good. We've already seen how the *size* of the brain enables us to have large social groups. It's also true that the *structure* of the brain is designed not so much for thinking as for relating to other people. In fact, you could conclude, as one writer did, that "the structure and function of the human brain is especially optimized for tasks that we would subsume under the heading of 'psychosocial competence.' Our brain is thus much more a social organ than it is a thinking organ."[6]

Studies show us too that compassion can be cultivated.[7] We are wired to relate to others and to respond to their needs, and we can grow in social competence and empathy. Just as I assure people that the only requirement to be a hospice volunteer is to show up, research shows that by being compassionate—by showing up, by thinking about others or by praying—we can develop a growing level of empathy for our neighbors.

One researcher discovered a number of activities that grow compassion among children. To the universal joy of parents, one of them is doing chores! In addition, parents who are responsive to children, play with them and simply touch them have been found to increase compassion among their children. Discussing compassion and acts of kindness also develops their empathy muscles, as does being with grandparents. Because the parts of the brain involved in compassion—in the frontal lobe—are still developing in a person's twenties, young people can make great growth in compassion into adulthood.[8]

The Neurons of Compassion

We are able to grow in compassion because the nerves that act as the "muscles of compassion" increase in effectiveness the more they operate. Humans, a few other primates and large whales all have the unique "von Economo neuron" residing in the brain's anterior cingulate, which sits behind the forehead. This special cell, also called a spindle neuron, is unusually large and can carry information across disparate areas of the brain. Scientists believe it is "intimately involved in the development of social awareness skills by integrating our thoughts, feelings, and behaviors."[9] These cells help guide us toward positive emotions.

The spindle cells sit in a place in the brain stimulated by prayer and contemplation. But this area is also exercised "whenever we see someone who is suffering, and this allows us to feel empathy and compassion."[10] In our brains, then, love for God and love for others are deeply intertwined.

On the other hand, stress, fear and anger shut off these compassion cells. Situations that produce fear and anxiety tend to shut down the areas of the brain involved in compassion and rational thinking. "When the amygdala [involved in feeling fear] becomes active, the anterior cingulate [compassion] shuts down. . . . Empathy and intuition decline, and you lose your ability to accurately assess how other people feel."[11]

Because of this, the fruits of the Spirit can serve as a very accurate assessment of a person's spiritual condition. When a person is generally quick to anger, judgmental or hateful, we can assume his or her anterior cingulate needs some exercise in prayer! On the other hand, someone full of joy, love, peace and kindness has trained the brain to respond to life with compassion.

The vagus nerve is another important component of the compassionate body. This set of cells runs from the brain down the spine to the organs of the stomach. It has a range of functions, including assisting in regulating speech, heart rate and blood pressure, and it conveys messages, including pain, from the organs to the brain. This nerve could be why we have "gut feelings" about people or situations.

University of California Berkeley professor Dacher Keltner calls the vagus a "caretaking organ" because it communicates with all the muscle groups that express compassion. For example, when a friend tells us about her troubles, we utter small sympathetic sighs. *Hmmm.* It is a natural and universal response that conveys to someone that we understand and sympathize with her suffering. "When we sigh in soothing fashion, or reassure others in distress with our concerned gaze or oblique eyebrows, the vagus nerve is doing its work." As the vagus nerve operates, it releases oxytocin, giving us a feeling of warmth and trust. When we get those good feelings by connecting with other people, our companions pick up on that feeling, sensing that we are deeply in tune with their state of emotions.[12]

When Keltner and other researchers measured the activity of volunteers' vagus nerves, they found that the more active a person's "caretaking organ" was, the more likely they were to have a substantial circle of friends and an active social life. They were more often seen to be warm and kind, upbeat and positive. They were seen to be more compassionate.

Interestingly, they were also more likely to experience awe. The ability to be moved by a beautiful sunset or a work of art is related to our experience of the divine. So when the researchers asked their subjects about experiences that had changed their sense of meaning and purpose, a number responded with stories of meaningful sermons, experiences of God and the sense that "God had a plan for me." Sixty-five percent of those with active vagus nerves had had such an experience in the three months between being tested and when they were asked about spiritual experiences. Not all experiences, of course, were Christian ones. Some were simply encounters with the natural world or moving lectures. However, a central theme of the spiritual experiences of those with active "caretaking organs" was that they tended to involve deeper connection to others, sacrifice and altruistic actions.[13]

The Chemical of Compassion

The vagus nerve doesn't only trigger facial muscles and soothing sounds that express our sympathy for another person. It also helps us to feel compassionate. The nerve is rich with oxytocin receptors, the chemical connected with our feelings of love and trust and empathy. "As the vagus nerve fires . . . presumably it triggers the release of oxytocin, sending signals of warmth, trust, and devotion throughout the brain and body and, ultimately, to other people."[14]

Of course our lives are more complex than this. We have periods of frustration and worry. In fact, as I learned in hospice, family caregivers may be bursting with oxytocin because they spend so much time caring for a loved one, but they also are heavily burdened, stressed and grieving the progressive loss of a once-mutual relationship. We may be naturally compassionate but be overwhelmed by financial stress, a destructive relationship, a difficult work environment or another source of stress outside of our control. We might have no say over these large factors, yet we can nudge ourselves in the direction of a more compassionate and peaceful orientation toward a fundamentally stressful situation.

Matthew Emerzian did just this. He was burned out working in the music industry, promoting bands like U2 and Coldplay, and one day began having panic attacks. They were serious enough that he eventually had to quit his job. He began seeing a therapist. She let him know that "the theme of [his] recovery was going to be, 'It's not about you.'"[15] She sent him every Saturday to feed the homeless, pick up trash or paint over graffiti. Acts of service became Matt's road back to health. After years of compassionate volunteering, Matt become a Christian and founded Every Monday Matters, an organization that encourages people to volunteer.[16]

Volunteering at a soup kitchen isn't a panacea, but little jolts of oxytocin serve an important purpose. Scientists have tried to measure the brain chemical in a controlled environment. In a series of experiments, scientists tried to measure college students' levels of oxytocin and their generosity and trust. In a money game commonly used to study economic behavior, the scientists gave two people the opportunity to share a large sum of money or for one person to hoard a smaller amount. The experimenter gives one person ten dollars, for example, and then asks the subject to share some with the other player. Whatever is shared, say five dollars, is then tripled and given to the second player. That player is then asked to share some with player number one.

This is a test of trust, because perfect self-interest would suggest that the first player would take the money and run. However, in a perfectly trusting environment, player one could share her whole gift with her companion, thereby tripling the total amount of money in the game. Player two would then split the total in half. In a perfectly trusting world, player number one would walk away with 50 percent more money.

Paul Zak and his colleagues measured the amount of money players trusted one another with and compared that to the level of oxytocin in their blood. What they found can probably be guessed at. Those who offered more money to other players had higher levels of oxytocin. Those who received money, and thereby felt trusted, also received jolts of oxytocin.

Then the researchers tried different versions of the experiment. If players received money by a clearly random process—and not a result of someone's trust—would they get the same boost in oxytocin? If they could artificially increase the amount of oxytocin in a person's bloodstream, would that person become more trusting? It turns out that random infusions of cash do nothing to increase the level of oxytocin. However, squirting oxytocin into a person's nose caused her or him to become extremely generous. Even massages boosted oxytocin levels and generosity. "As for cause and effect, we found that we could turn the behavioral response on and off like a garden hose."[17]

These experiments simply show us one key aspect in a complex system. Understanding how oxytocin or the compassion nerves work is like knowing how a light switch or the transformer on the electrical line works. They are important parts of a much more complex electrical system that includes electric utility companies, power plants and a web of power lines and station. Our own biological system of compassion integrates our brains, our peripheral nervous system by way of our vagus nerves, our facial muscles, vocal cords and other body expressions, plus neurochemicals that gives us the feeling of warm compassion, trust and attachment to other people. Through this complex biology, we recognize another person's needs and respond to them, from a simple *Hmm* in a conversation to mission trips and lifestyles of service.

The Emotions of the Good Life

The good Samaritan is the poster child for compassion. Without thought to his reputation or pocketbook, he stops to care for a wounded man along the road. Going beyond the call of duty, he transports the man to a place where he can recover and pays for his care. Luke tells us very little about the good Samaritan's state of mind as he performed this kind act of service. All that we know is that the good Samaritan took pity on the wounded man (Lk 10:33).

Brain systems aren't merely physiological tools. They enable us to express ourselves to other people and to be understood, to give and receive compassion. In them we see the design of a loving God. So we can assume that the good Samaritan's emotions directed his behaviors. His feelings of pity moved him to service as oxytocin flooded his brain, prompting him to go the extra mile to love his neighbor. This same pattern can be a regular part of our spiritual experiences as we, like the good Samaritan, seek to care for those with whom we come into contact.

Of course we can be selfish, inconsiderate and cruel to others, but these aren't the emotions that produce meaningful, joyful and happy lives. Studies show that happiness and joy over a lifetime always result from acting compassionately toward other people.[18] The best way to pursue your own joy is to join a church, volunteer in your community, care for the needy, raise a family or pursue life in community. Chasing after our own pleasure can affect short-term happiness but does not lead to long-term joy and peace. As we connect to God, we also tend to change how we understand ourselves, shifting from self-centeredness toward the welfare of others.

We discover who we are in relation to others. We meet our own deepest needs by caring for those around us. We find happiness when we make others happy. From the muscles around our eyes that make us squint when we smile to the visceral reaction in our gut when we see suffering, our bodies are designed to express our own needs and compassion as well as to respond to the needs of others. We don't have two levels of relationships, one horizontal with others and one vertical with God. The two are inextricably linked.

This is why practically nobody plays the trust game as economic theory would predict. Few people can actually take the money and run. We share because money and the things it can buy cannot make us happy. What drives us isn't collecting stuff but connecting to others and compassionately responding to their needs. "The emotions that promote the meaningful life are organized according to an interest in the welfare of others," says one researcher.[19] Because our own enjoyment in life is linked to others, we learn to turn our attention outward. We shift our idea of who we are and what we love away from purely personal objectives and toward the needs we discover as we relate to other people. And at the promptings of our faith, we may even go so far as the good Samaritan and respond when we see our political enemy wounded by the side of the road.

After telling the story of the good Samaritan, Jesus asks his listener who acted as a neighbor to the wounded man, and the expert in the law responds with no hesitation: the man who performed acts of service is the neighbor. Jesus' response? "Go and do likewise."

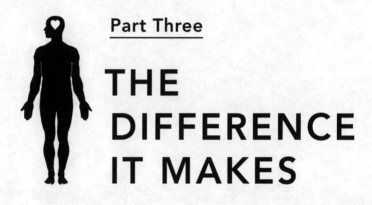

Part Three

THE
DIFFERENCE
IT MAKES

10

NEURO-TRANSFORMATION

IN THE 1970S MY YOUNG-ADULT PARENTS tried to turn on, tune in and drop out with their fellow hippies, but they quickly became disillusioned. They were searching for something deeper, and they found it in a vibrant group of Christians meeting in the basement of a YMCA in the Rogers Park neighborhood of Chicago. They turned on to Jesus.

In that basement my parents met a group of people who were much like them, disenchanted hippies who wanted to pursue a new kind of love. Many were leaving drugs and the rest of the counterculture. As they grew in their newfound faith, they routinely burned the trappings of the old ways of life, from records to bellbottoms. Sometimes these were replaced and then burned again. A number of their new friends had grown up in church and rejected it as stale and irrelevant. So as they returned to God, they were not interested in joining any ordinary church. They sought a countercultural revolution modeled on the book of Acts.

Powered by the gospel, my parents and their friends formed a community of intense prayer and praise that extended from all day Sunday through the rest of the week, with prayer meetings, small group meetings, Bible studies, community dinners and outreach gatherings. Church services began on the sidewalk outside the building as worshipers were gathering together. It was a world where the Spirit of God moved, healed, breathed and transformed lives.

Eventually these "Jesus freaks" settled into jobs and suburban mortgages, but they still practiced an intense, relational Christianity. Wednesday-night prayer meetings included no preaching, simply an hour and a half or two hours of constant prayer. Sometimes few requests were given, and the hours were spent praying Scripture or the poetry of hymn texts. Prayers were offered for the souls of coworkers, neighbors and friends. Outside of church, members called one another and prayed over the phone.

Stories of lives profoundly changed by the gospel surrounded me as I grew up. These believers had gotten off drugs and given up wild lifestyles. It seemed as if everyone had a testimony of dramatic transformation through Jesus. When I, or my church kid friends, would complain that we also wanted these powerful experiences of personal change, we always heard the same response: we should be glad we didn't carry the baggage of an old way of life. While meeting Jesus had launched them on their new lives, change was hard.

Christians tend to separate salvation into two distinct processes—the "easy work" of simply requiring an acceptance of Jesus' gift of new life and the "hard work" of sanctification, the working out of that salvation. However, neither is really easy. The step of faith and personal change are equally arduous, but the spiritual process of becoming more like Christ is made possible physically in part by prayer, worship and other spiritual experiences. Moments when we meet with God are powerful catalysts for personal change. As the emotional intensity of a spiritual experience increases, the existing neural connections in our brain become unstable, allowing for the creation of new connections, new ideas and new understandings of oneself and the world. Very quickly, transformation becomes quite possible (and with powerful experiences inevitable) as our neurons develop new connections.[1]

As Christians, we live into our new nature to shed our old ways and grow into the likeness of Christ. Our brains are always changing based on new experiences and new information. Neurons form new "arms" called dendrites and axons and connect to one another, making physical changes in the brain that allow us to recall a memory or information. Change doesn't come easily, but as we establish new patterns of thinking and habits, the neural pathways that were once new and difficult grow firmer and more well traveled.

These neurological patterns are essential so that we don't require intense concentration for frequent activities. We need to be able to drive, for example, without having to think about whether the accelerator is on the right or the left or to bring to mind the name and landmarks of every street. But when those pathways are unhealthy or do not change as we mature, then they can be destructive. Thankfully, connection to God can make those pathways susceptible to change.

The science of neuroplasticity explains how every experience changes the brain, but it also shows that most lasting transformation comes by intentional and attentive training. It shows how prayer, study and community would have changed people like my parents from groovy hippies into churchgoing prayer warriors.

Brain Plasticity

For decades, scientists believed that once the brain was developmentally mature it was basically set in stone. Different areas of the brain were responsible for different functions, it was believed, so that damage to a given area would forever destroy the abilities associated with that region. Conventional wisdom held that new brain cells didn't grow and that injury to the brain, such as by a stroke, caused permanent damage. Brains were like teeth: you had to work with the ones you got.

But within the past couple of decades, the notion of the fixed brain has been overturned. Brains not only are surprisingly adaptable but are actually changing all the time. Disorders and diseases of the brain, even strokes that kill massive numbers of brain cells, can be treated or compensated for.

An astounding set of experiments show that the brain is capable of drastically rearranging itself based on our experience. In one of the studies that broke open the debate on whether the brain can change, a scientist was able to teach a blind person to process visual signals from a video camera.

Because our eyes simply translate light into neural impulses, Paul Bach-y-Rita thought he might be able to teach a blind person to see by providing a different source that would produce the same neural impulses as an eye. He was able to set up a video camera attached to a tactile pad that covered merely a ten-inch square area of skin on a blind subject's back. The pad represented the scene on the camera through an array of raised pressure points. After just a few hours, the subject's brain figured out that the tactile impressions on his back were not a massage but visual input. His brain then was able to translate that input into images that the subject was able to see. It became possible for the patient to make out objects and make his way around a room thanks to the scene displayed on his back. (Maybe having eyes on the back of one's head isn't so far-fetched!)[2]

The device has since been refined so that a blind person can wear sunglasses with a camera on them. The camera transmits signals onto a device on the tongue that transmits tiny electrical signals to the brain, which then reads the signals as sight. Patients don't have perfect vision with the device, but they can find their way around an unfamiliar environment or learn to decipher letters. An Iraq war veteran who lost his sight due to a rocket-propelled grenade was able to make out letters on an optical test. "It was amazing," he told a British newspaper. "Then I walked down a corridor and I could make out the doorways, the walls and people coming towards me."[3]

If our brains didn't change, a blind person's huge visual cortex would be useless. Instead, with the tactile pad the brain uses the visual cortex in a different way, learning to pick up visual signals from the skin on the back instead of light bouncing off the retina. It also means that the skin's nerve cells rewire to send their signals to the areas of the brain involved in sight rather than areas involved in processing touch.

In a similar kind of experiment on ferrets, researchers switched the nerves connecting the auditory and visual processing centers shortly after birth. The part of the ferret's brain that normally received input from the ears was forced to process sight. While the auditory part of the brain did not see perfectly, the ferrets' sight was good enough to show that the brain could be retrained to process information differently. It was one of the first incontrovertible pieces of evidence that the brain wires and rewires itself according to experience. "It's about the most compelling demonstration you could have that experience shapes the brain," said one researcher.[4]

Since these and other experiments began showing that the brain is not a static organ, researchers have applied their discoveries to stroke victims and others who suffer brain damage, even mentally disabled children and people who suffer from obsessive-compulsive disorder. They have found that even people with massive damage to the brain can relearn lost skills as the brain reengineers itself, rewires neurons and learns new skills.

How the Brain Changes

We say that the brain is "plastic" because any learning requires billions of neurons to make physical changes that enable them to better connect to one another. The brain is made up of around 100 billion neurons, each of which is connected to a thousand other neurons. This gives the brain about 100 trillion connections between neurons. The brain is therefore an incredibly complex organ, perhaps one of the most complex things in the universe.

The complexity of the brain becomes mind-blowing when you consider that each of the 100 trillion connections between neurons can have various states. Computers have binary signals, 1s and 0s, on and off, as their basic signaling device. In the neural connections in our brains, there may be ten or more possible states between two neurons. This is why the brain is called the most complex thing in existence. There are more potential brain states than there are particles in the universe. Simply understanding how the brain processes vision—with some neurons dedicated to processing movement, others to color, others to shapes, others to faces—is a task well beyond current science.

When cells communicate, they do so through a mix of electrical and chemical signals. Those signals can change, increase and decrease in strength, or develop from scratch. One cell receives signals from another through its dendrites, branches with ports capable of picking up a chemical signal from another neuron. Having received a signal, the dendrites send an electrical impulse up their branches into the body of the cell and then out through one or more of their many axons. At the tip of the axon is the synapse, the space between one dendrite and the dendrites of the next cell. The various signals a cell might send or receive can be strong or weak, and a neuron can amplify or weaken the signal it received.

Much of the growth and development occurs in our synapses as we learn. The axon will send a chemical signal across the synapse to the dendrites of the next neuron. Most medications that affect mood and behavior have their impact at this point by either increasing or decreasing the chemicals available here. When we talk about brain chemicals such as dopamine or endorphins, this is where they come into play.

Using these neurotransmitters, cells communicate, and their ability to communicate increases the more they work together. The chemical signals sent from one side of the synapse become stronger, and the receptors on the other side become more sensitive, better able to pick up signals. As we learn a new activity or new information or even a new dance step, neurons are making new connections at new synapses and strengthening others.

The brain does more than receive input from the body and process it. The brain is always on the move, so to speak, improving how it processes information and searching for new information. It is learning and learning how to learn. Our brains will employ a host of neurons to allow us to learn something new, but as we gain in proficiency, fewer cells are needed, which then become more specialized in doing their task. They fuse more tightly. They create neural pathways.

Experience is constantly changing our brains. The cerebral cortex—the wrinkled outer layer of the brain involved in high-level thinking—is 5 percent heavier in laboratory mammals that receive mental training or learning enriched environments. Rats who are trained on difficult special problems have higher levels of acetyl-choline, a chemical necessary for learning, in their brains. Neurons in those stimulated regions grow larger, developing 25 percent more branches, more connections to other neurons. Because of their extra work, they even demand more blood supply. Examinations of human brains after death shows that people with more education tend to have literally bigger brains.[5] Cells can grow new connections with other neurons, often more than doubling their integration with other cells. This physical learning process often means that learning something new doesn't require forgetting something old. By increasing the brain's synaptic connections, we can also increase its capacity.

The brain is in many ways like a muscle, growing stronger the more it gets used. It has a basic structure or mode of operations. But within that framework the brain is surprisingly flexible, even into old age and even after the diseases of old age hamper its function. While the extreme but necessary neural nimbleness of youth is lost shortly after adolescence, the ability of the brain to change and grow throughout life is only now being understood.

This should come as encouragement to us; we are not set in stone. We can and do change dramatically. But the change that occurs naturally over time we can make happen on our own. Researchers have been looking at how to create the brain changes that we desire.

Principles for Transformation

The brain is a conservative organ. It does only what it must, so there are certain conditions required for a plastic change. First, we must pay close attention. We do not change our brains while surfing the Internet, flipping stations or monitoring Facebook. In numerous experiments, researchers found that while neurons will change as a result of inattentive experience, they revert to their original state shortly after. Changing who we are requires the kind of attention that many of us have not exerted since we last needed arithmetic flashcards.

In spiritual practices, the attention required in deep prayer and contemplation, study or worship is what the brain needs to grow and enhance neural connections. Andrew Newberg found that after eight weeks of meditation, he has been able to measure changes in the brain. It can take just two weeks, and sometimes even less time, for neurons to grow new axons and dendrites, making new connections to other neurons and making new learning a physical feature of the brain.[6]

Newberg also found that this kind of spiritual practice is unique in the way it changes the brain. Any kind of learning, and any kind of concentration, will cause the brain to change in response. "But religious and spiritual contemplation changes your brain in a profoundly different way because it strengthens a unique neural circuit that specifically enhances social awareness and empathy while subduing destructive feelings and emotions."[7] That's what makes spirituality particularly healthy for your brain.

Finally, the emotional nature of spiritual experiences helps us to change as well. Prayer and other spiritual practices like worship are more than cognitive exercises. Feeling close to God is emotionally powerful, and those emotions can create neural instability. The connections between neurons loosen up, allowing new connections to form. As an example of the kind of spiritual experience that can produce this kind of change, Newberg points to "hitting bottom" for an addict, when she or he fully recognizes dependency and submits to God and others for help. Newberg says, "There is no doubt that heightened emotionality in a context of surrender increases the possibility of self-transformation."[8]

When Saul met the Lord on the Damascus Road, this is precisely what happened to him. A powerful supernatural encounter provided the heightened emotionality. Acts 9 tells us Saul fell to the ground trembling and astonished when he saw the bright light and heard the voice of Christ. If that wasn't enough to convince Saul away from his former life, God caused him to become blind—a very physical surrendering of his natural abilities. Dumbfounded by this meeting with the Lord, the blind Saul had to be led by the hand into Damascus by his companions (Acts 9:8). The Scriptures tell us that during his days of blindness Saul neither ate not drank. Whether this response resulted simply from the shock of his experience or whether Saul was prompted to fast, his divine encounter was already producing within him the transformation that God desired.

For whatever reason, though, we don't all get to have dramatic experiences. We experience God in quiet moments as we read Scripture, gather in church, pray, meet in small groups with other Christians or simply take a walk in the woods. And for these more serene encounters to add up to a life that is directed in love for God and others, we must exert intentional effort.

Strengthening the Spiritual Circuit

This intentional effort is seen most dramatically in the cases of stroke victims working hard to relearn basic skills. Their attention and intensive practice of even the most mundane tasks like picking up a fork or walking show us that concerted effort can strengthen the circuits necessary for real, measurable change. Edward Taub, a plasticity researcher who works with such victims, says his experience shows that for success, this kind of focused learning is necessary. We don't learn while multitasking, and we don't learn casually.

To change our brains and therefore ourselves, we must train ourselves to do simple tasks over and over again. Taub's stroke clinic makes use of the kind of repetitive training we usually see only in movies, dramatically highlighted and fast-forwarded—the running back who practices by charging up a steep dirt hill over and over again, the martial artist practicing moves over and over again or the spelling bee competitor memorizing obscure words. For the stroke victim in Taub's clinic, that might mean picking up a bean and putting it in a bowl over and over again. It might mean turning a doorknob and pushing a door open again and again.

In addition, "training should be done in increments; and work should be concentrated into a short time."[9] Taub calls this technique "massed practice." Where typical stroke rehab involves therapy for a couple of hours a few days a week, Taub's patients work all day long for two full weeks. His patients master a skill that is only incrementally more difficult than what they can already do. Then they move on to the next step, but they must constantly work at it. Taub's "massed practice," like language immersion, forces the learner to quickly make and solidify the new neural connections necessary to developing the new skill.

What his research, and the experience of his patients, shows is that even when the brain has experienced massive damage, it can recruit healthy cells to do what the damaged ones can no longer do. With the right method, we can choose to radically rewire our brains.

Spiritual practices combine all these ingredients: attention, emotion and even massed practice. In his book *Prayer: Does It Make Any Difference?* Philip Yancey writes that his fellow author Brennan Manning told him that no one had ever failed to hear from God during one of the retreats Manning had led. There were just a few expectations for the retreat, including worship and some guidance from Manning, but the one rule was to spend two hours a day in prayer.

Taub's research on neural plasticity can help us to better understand why this happens with such regularity. We often assume that feelings of devotion must inspire our daily prayer or devotional time. If we pray and don't "feel" that God showed up, it's hard to keep going. But what if we could grow more and more like Christ, knowing that our daily faithful habits were building that relationship piece by piece? The knowledge of how our bodies are designed could provide the inspiration to keep trying, even when the work seems arduous. Taub's research explains how so many people like my parents changed from hippies who tuned out into Jesus freaks who were intensely tuned in, praying for hours in a single sitting. Prayer changes things, as they say, including your brain.

The various ways we practice knowing God involve these techniques. When we pray, study, meditate on Scripture, we focus our attention, and we slowly develop our ability to connect with God. Many people find prayer and contemplation methods to be hard. We sit down to pray, and nothing happens. We try to find God, but he isn't there. The same is true for the stroke victim who can't use his left arm. But as he puts mental effort into the attempt, slowly he can do what was once impossible. When a woman sits down to pray and finds it impossible, that very effort, when repeated again and again, makes possible what was once impossible.

Studying God

While the hippies were on their quest for self-discovery, Kent Schnake was getting his degree in engineering at Carnegie Mellon University and then his master's at Cornell. While the hippies were discovering the things of the Spirit in the Age of Aquarius, Kent had decided that there was no God. Even as a child, he never went to church. "Early on," he says, "I bought into a secular materialist worldview." In fact, during high school he would find Christians and argue with them, using all the reasons that vociferous opponents of religion, like Richard Dawkins, might use today. Landing a job at Hewlett Packard put Kent at a place, he says, where most of this colleagues shared his worldview.

During his mid-twenties, Kent's assurance about the material universe began to crumble. His marriage was in trouble, and through counseling, Kent recognized that he had been abusing drugs and alcohol to deal with crippling anxiety. While his marriage continued to unravel, Kent's therapist suggested she was not the person to help him with anxiety. She referred Kent to a psychiatrist, who prescribed benzodiazepines, which are prescribed today in the form of Valium or Xanax.

From there, Kent's life went from bad to worse. His marriage ended, and he gave in to a destructive, self-centered lifestyle. Kent began abusing his medication, mixing it with illegal drugs and alcohol. "I just wanted to run wild," Kent told me. He had felt trapped by his marriage. "So I very selfishly decided it wasn't working for me, and the only way to get out was to end it. When I did that, I really had a lot of time on my hands and even less center and direction. So what I did was party. I went out drinking a lot."

Kent continued to earn good money at his job, but all of his spare time he wasted on drugs and partying. By this point in his life, in his early thirties, Kent had begun to see a number of cracks in the godless materialist worldview he held. He continued to mask his anxiety with drugs, and those drugs began to conflict with his life.

After Kent remarried, he and his wife had their first child—a wakeup call for Kent, who realized he didn't want to raise that baby in the partying and drug environment in which he was living. He also recognized that he needed some sense of meaning and purpose in his life. He began keeping a journal in which he wondered about life and how to create meaning. Kent now considered himself agnostic rather than an atheist. The journal was a way of paying attention to his life and questions, an exercise that many use to deepen their faith.[10]

Finally, Kent took a few steps to get his life under control. He and his new wife moved to Oregon to find a more rural setting to raise their family and—hopefully—to kick Kent's drinking habit. But Kent found that change wasn't easy. Even in a new place, "you find new people to drink with, people to buy drugs from," he explained. For some of his drugs, though, Kent needed a prescription, and that meant that he needed to find a new doctor.

The first doctor Kent visited didn't make it easy to get what he wanted. "He asked me some questions," Kent said, "and I think I answered pretty truthfully, and consequently he said, 'You're an alcoholic and you're addicted to these drugs, so I'm not going to give you any. But I will help you quit.'" To hear his problem stated so bluntly, Kent says, was what he needed to get serious about addressing his addiction.

One of the treatments Kent's psychiatrist prescribed was to go to church and develop a spiritual life. The doctor wasn't a Christian, but he recognized the value of spirituality in helping someone quit drugs and alcohol. He recommended a church simply because it was easy for his patients to find the support they needed at a church.

Kent found a Pentecostal church that he liked, and while he still didn't believe in God, he appreciated that the church was serious about its beliefs and that the people were honestly working on developing a spiritual life. He spent time expanding his spiritual horizons reading the psychologist William James and the psychotherapist Carl Jung. Neither had much use for an objective, external God, but both respected spiritual experience as a personal and emotional fact.

Slowly, through intentional work like journaling, focused reading and church attendance, Kent's views of God were shifting, and he was staying off drugs and alcohol. But it was another decision he made that forever changed his life. He began getting up a half-hour early every morning to focus on his spiritual life and his attempt to change. "I wanted to clear up my concept of God," he says.

No longer an atheist or even an agnostic, Kent felt he needed to figure out what he thought of God. He began reading a Bible he had been given, as well as a Christian book, during his morning half-hour. As Kent tells the story, this was a very cerebral exercise, mentally pondering his questions about God and not really praying or meditating. Still, this kind of study involves focused attention, the kind necessary for personal change.

Quitting drugs and alcohol had given him a deep sense of humility, Kent says. They were making him feel horrible when he was on them, but leaving them behind was physically grueling. "I had this motivation and humiliation to think about how I was going to fill up that void," he says. Kent was primed for surrender, and unknowingly he was creating new neural pathways that would enable him to connect with God.

One morning during his study, Kent felt God speak to him. "He said to me, 'I'm not your concept; you are my concept.'" It inverted how Kent had been thinking about God. "All of a sudden it was about what God thought of me, not what I thought of him. 'How did he make me?' rather than how I made him up." Kent dropped to the floor, got on his knees and began to pray.

"From that point on," Kent says, "I attended church and considered myself born again. I took it very seriously. I had set out to find purpose in life. I found there was. Now I was serious about building on that."

Kent's quest to get off drugs and alcohol had led him on a spiritual journey that brought him to a profound experience of God. That experience helped him further along the road of recovery. Plenty of people kick bad habits without prayer, but for Kent as well as for many others, recognizing God's place in his life—discovering he was God's creation, not the other way around—helped him to find the strength in his own weakness that he needed to overcome his addictions.

Over the years, Kent's life changed dramatically. Now one of his children is a missionary, and Kent uses his business skills to help her mission agency. He has discovered a new purpose for his life in retirement, encouraging people who are mentally ill. His heart for this ministry may come in part from the fact that anxiety is still a part of his life. It is something Kent has learned to manage through prayer and other techniques, but it remains as a challenge for him, a "thorn" God has chosen not to remove.

Through prayer, worship and study, as God rewires our brains and renews our minds, he makes us into new creatures. We can allow God to work his change in our lives by intentionally pursuing encounters with him. Our brains are made to change and to learn based on our experiences and our own efforts. Traditional spiritual practices seem to be rooted in the facts that modern science is only now discovering about how brains change. When we give focused attention and regular practice, whether through prayer, study, meditation, journaling or other means of attending to the presence of God, we can experience God in profound ways that lead to permanent changes in our lives.

THE GREAT PHYSICIAN

IN 2006, RESEARCHERS HELD A NEWS CONFERENCE announcing the results of the most expensive, largest and longest study ever on the effectiveness of prayer on healing. Herbert Benson, a Harvard researcher and doctor who has straddled the worlds of Western scientific medicine and alternative therapies, served as a lead on the study. Benson has argued for and conducted research on the effectiveness of prayer in improving a person's health. Through his research and writings, Benson has popularized prayer and meditation as a scientifically based technique for treating everything from high blood pressure to pain and insomnia.

The study cost $2.4 million to fund and involved eighteen hundred patients at six hospitals. It used the most rigorous analytical methods a study like this can employ, randomly assigning some patients for prayer, others for no prayer, and ensuring that those praying as well as the patients were blinded to one another. The researchers successfully isolated prayer as the only variable that could explain any potential differences between the health of the groups of patients who were studied. Three Christian religious communities agreed to pray for patients just prior to surgery and to continue to do so between one and four times for the next fourteen days.[1]

The results of previous studies had not been entirely conclusive. Some had suggested prayer was helpful to the sick, while others suggested it made no difference. Yet there were tantalizing indications that an ambitious study like this would finally answer the question, is prayer effective in treating illness?

When the study was finally released, however, the authors—as well as others who have promoted the healing effects of prayer—began backpedaling. Perhaps a massive study was not the way to study prayer. From the beginning, researchers offered explanations for the study's failure. "This study might be opening doors to show the power of mind-body interventions both positively and negatively," said Benson.[2]

The results showed that those who received prayer actually did worse than those who did not, and the patients who knew they were being prayed for did the worst. The study found "complications occurred in 52% (315/604) of patients who received intercessory prayer versus 51% (304/597) of those who did not." Both groups were told that they might or might not receive prayer. However, patients who were told that someone would certainly be praying for them did the worst. Compared to just over half of the other groups, 59 percent of patients who knew they were being prayed for had complications. According to the study, "certainty of receiving intercessory prayer was associated with a higher incidence of complications."[3]

Those who study health and spirituality were unable to prove that intercessory prayer would conclusively benefit patients' health. Instead, they suggested that such a study might never show scientific proof. "The problem with studying religion scientifically is that you do violence to the phenomenon by reducing it to basic elements that can be quantified, and that makes for bad science and bad religion," said Richard Sloan, Nathaniel Wharton Professor of Behavioral Medicine at Columbia University.[4]

Despite the data in this study, other experts in the field hold firm to their conviction that prayer and healing may be connected. Harold Koenig at Duke University said, "I think that prayer absolutely does work and that God answers prayer and that we can continue to pray for our loved ones. We should not think that science can answer every question there is."[5]

In an email interview, Koenig explained why such studies are bound to fail but also why he believes prayer does indeed produce healing. "These studies are worthless from both a scientific and a theological standpoint. If they did show something (consistently), then this would suggest that God is part of the created universe, since it is possible to control God's actions and measure them in a scientific study." Koenig said that intercessory prayer studies mostly serve the interests of "New Agers who believe in telepathy and psychokinesis" who are looking to show that thoughts or prayer can have effects in the material world. These areas, says Koenig, "have no scientific credibility whatsoever." Nevertheless, Koenig's extensive research on prayer, spiritual practices and healing shows conclusively that prayer is indeed effective, and it can be measured so long as researchers look at prayer and spirituality within a holistic framework that includes a religious community.

Putting spiritual experience into a laboratory can empty spiritual practice of its content. Some of these studies, for example, separate those praying and those being prayed for, or they require specific prayers to be said in order to control as many variables as possible. Candy Gunther Brown, a professor at Indiana University who studies the healing effects of prayer, writes that such studies lack "construct validity." In other words, they fail to understand what believers find to be effective in prayer. By using the methods used for pharmaceutical drug trials, researchers aren't studying prayer so much as the effects of the mutterings of distant strangers. "Lack of theological understanding by researchers," says Brown, "has meant that even if intercessory prayer, as it is most often practiced contextually, 'works,' most study designs would likely not be able to find existing empirical effects, because they do not isolate the prayer phenomena that practitioners claim to be effective."[6]

As Christians, we believe with Harold Koenig that prayer works. The apostle James exhorts believers to pray for those who are sick or in trouble. He even asserts that prayers offered for a sick person will bring healing, because "the prayer of a righteous person is powerful and effective" (Jas 5:16). Yet for all of the prayers for healing that we see answered in the here and now, there are many more that seem to go unanswered, or are answered in ways we would not choose. To understand the intersection of our faith and bodily life, we must explore how our health is affected by spiritual practices. Our health, or lack of it, can be a place where we meet with God and connect deeply with him.

Effective Prayer

Our faith has a remarkable effect on our bodies, even if Benson's study showed that the prayers of distant strangers don't have much effect. Those who are close to the work of healing believe that prayer certainly does have a positive effect on health. One survey found that 94 percent of executives at HMOs (health maintenance organizations) believe prayer helps medical treatment and speeds the recovery of patients. Another survey found that nearly three-quarters of doctors believe in miraculous healings.[7]

So while researchers cannot find the link between prayer and health, the overwhelming majority of practitioners believe such a link exists. They confirm the beliefs of most Americans, 23 percent of whom say they have witnessed divine healing of someone's health troubles. In 2003 a study found that 72 percent of Americans believed that "praying to God can cure someone—even if science says the person doesn't stand a chance."[8]

While the specific link between intercessory prayer and health is unclear, clearly that uncertainty has not changed the views of medical experts that praying for others makes a difference. They believe, along with the population generally, that prayer matters.

While *specific prayers* for health haven't been scientifically linked to better health, *praying* and spiritual practices have. Science has made that abundantly clear. The connection is so strong that, as some researchers write, "lack of religious involvement has an effect on mortality that is equivalent to forty years of smoking one pack of cigarettes per day."[9]

There have been well over a thousand studies on the relationship between religion and spirituality and health.[10] Those studies conclude that worship, prayer, going to church and holding positive beliefs about God (that all things work together for good, for example, as opposed to beliefs that God is punishing the sick) are like eating your vegetables. Faith, like a regular dose of leafy greens, isn't a "wonder drug," but it does prod us toward better health. Between 1992 and 2006 the number of medical schools that offered courses on religion, spirituality and medicine increased from 3 to 141, as health care professionals are learning make use of faith's powerful health effects. Not only are the courses offered, but 70 percent of them are required.[11]

A person's beliefs and spiritual practices have a significant effect even when they don't change the outcome of her or his health. One study found that patients who told researchers that they did not receive spiritual support cost $2,441 more for care in their last week of life than patients who said their spiritual needs were met.

In addition, patients who relied on their faith to help deal with their health decline cost slightly less than the average patient. However, among patients who relied on their faith, costs were 174 percent greater ($6,395 vs. $2,335) when their spiritual needs were *not* met compared to those who felt supported spiritually. Aside from intercessory prayer studies, faith clearly has a huge impact on our health.[12]

When we consider these numbers, two ideas seem evident. First, we shouldn't expect scientific research to be able to investigate the will of God. When God chooses to miraculously intervene in someone's health problem, we must respond simply with praise. Even the most sophisticated research techniques cannot chart the hand of God.

Second, if God has indeed created us to love him and to love our neighbors, the practices that are involved in cultivating a love for God and in serving our neighbors ought to be good for us. They go along with the nature of the world God has created. As Koenig said to me in an email, "The 'owner's manual' (the Bible) tells us how to live, believe, and treat others. When we do what it says, health is the result. I'd say that objective research supports that." There are real material benefits to walking with the Lord, even in broken bodies still longing for ultimate transformation.

Religious Pathways of Health

In his book *Medicine, Religion, and Health: Where Science and Spirituality Meet*, Koenig says that while science can't investigate the will of God, it is "capable of looking at natural explanations. Therefore, the most obvious and plausible 'natural' way that religion might impact physical health is through pathways that are psychological, social, and behavioral."[13] While scientists can't measure the divine, they can measure the impact of joining a church and receiving support from that church. Science can measure the health impact of feeling at peace and living a meaningful life. While these effects aren't "miraculous," we should fully appreciate how positive the effects of faith and religious practice are on our health.

Religion's effect on our behavior is clear. When religious norms discourage drinking, immoral behavior and gambling, for obvious reasons it results in better health. Exhortations like Paul's "Do not get drunk on wine" (Eph 5:18) produce clear health results, yet there is no proof of the divine in them. It doesn't take a miracle to experience the health impact of getting sober.

We may not see measurable evidence of the power of the Holy Spirit when a drinking father cleans up his life, settles into a job and spends more time with his family. Yet as in Kent Schnake's case, we shouldn't discount the significance of such a turnaround and the spiritual power that enables it and is produced by it. Once when I visited the work of a humanitarian organization in Cambodia, a local fisherman freely admitted to me that he had been a terrible husband and father and a heavy drinker. Needing a better income, he sought the help of a microfinance agency that taught him money management skills such as budgeting and saving. They directed the fisherman toward more profitable employment. More important, he said, they taught him discipline. As the fisherman worked harder, his income grew, and more of it went toward helping his family. Because it was a Christian microfinance institution that was helping him, he slowly became interested in joining the church. Soon his family became Christians.

This father's lifestyle turnaround will have long-term health consequences. Better income and finances will reduce stress and possibly allow him to afford medical care should he need it. And getting off alcohol will be good for his liver and bring good effects in a host of other areas of his life and that of his whole family. But this was not simply a physical transformation. It was also clearly a spiritual one, miraculous in a different way from a healing from cancer or the blind receiving sight. Becoming a Christian was only the latest step of the work of the Holy Spirit enabling and making a dissolute father willing to change his life.

Spirituality encourages people toward a healthy lifestyle, but that isn't the only "pathway" by which faith affects our health. As we have seen, social interactions affect the very nature of who we are. And that is especially true of our connections to people at church and others who share our faith.

For example, researchers have found that "positive social interactions and psychological states may boost immune, endocrine, and cardiovascular functions, thereby protecting against disease or slowing its progression."[14] In addition, volunteering and other altruistic social behavior have been found to improve psychological and physical health.[15]

Positive relationships can make it much easier to deal with illness when a person has a group of family and friends to rely on for support. On the whole, religious people tend to have stronger social networks, encouraging altruistic behavior. But church-based relationships have been found to have greater health effects than other relationships. One study found that "church membership was the only type of social involvement that predicted greater life satisfaction and happiness."[16] Another study found that church-based friendships were the only social factor that predicted life satisfaction.[17] (Researchers distinguish between happiness and satisfaction. You can be happy day to day and dissatisfied with your life, or unhappy because of overwhelming day-to-day challenges and yet be satisfied with your life.)

Koenig concludes, "Not only is religious involvement associated with higher social support, the health effects of church-related support appear to be greater than the effects of support obtained outside of the church. Recent research confirms these reports."[18] Why are church-based relationships so powerful? It may be because we invest greater meaning in them. These relationships are the places where we care for others or receive care. We aren't just doing something kind; we are behaving as God has called us to do.

Removing the Stress Effect

Faith's behavioral and social "pathways" affect health. So too does faith influence our psychology. Since the brain regulates all the body's systems and every area of the brain is intertwined with the rest, how we feel affects our health.

Herbert Benson, the author of the inconclusive prayer study, was among the first to identify the psychological link between thoughts and health and popularize a therapy to exploit it. In his bestselling book *The Relaxation Response*, Benson argues that many modern diseases can be caused or complicated by stress: high blood pressure and heart ailments, depression and anxiety, cough and cold sores, infertility and insomnia, pain and arthritis, as well as side effects of cancer and AIDS.[19] A long list of diseases could be successfully treated not with medicine, surgery or doctor visits, he argues, but rather by the calming effects that result from prayer.

Benson teaches a thoroughly secular method of eliciting the relaxation response, but he also shows that it is only an adaptation of the kind of prayer practiced in many religions. Benson spends twelve pages of his short book exploring Christian teaching on prayer from Martin Luther and medieval mystics to early Orthodox fathers. He writes that 80 percent of his patients choose to pray when practicing the relaxation response. While 80 percent pray, roughly 25 percent of his patients say they feel more spiritual because of it.[20]

That sense of closeness to God has an added health effect. While the calming effect of the ritual is important, Benson says that feeling connected to God makes an even bigger difference. Those who described themselves as feeling more spiritual had "fewer medical symptoms than do those who reported no increase in spirituality from the elicitation."[21]

Benson wrote that modern life tends to activate our fight-or-flight reflex. Driving in heavy traffic, the stresses of work and other demands of modern life regularly activate a state of high anxiety. Since we rarely ever actually fight or flee, we also never have the opportunity to come down from this restless state. The buildup of stress does not get released, and we are subject to the resulting ill health effects.

Stress causes far more health problems than just hypertension. Benson says, "Studies indicate that between 60 and 90 percent of all our population's visits to doctors' offices" are because of the effects of stress. As much as 74 percent of complaints brought to medical clinics cannot be traced to specific physical sources "and are probably caused by 'psychosocial' factors." For this reason, Benson believes that most of the treatment offered in those clinics is ineffective. The only hope a patient has to heal comes from her or his own bodily mechanisms.[22] Seventy-four percent is an astonishingly high figure. Consider for a moment your own medical visits or just the odd pains here and there that have annoyed you through the last few years. When we visit the doctor, we tend to look to him or her for answers about our ailments. But if Benson's numbers are accurate, our bodies perhaps could heal themselves, if given the opportunity. Benson's point is not to discredit the advice of physicians. After all, he is a cardiologist by training. Instead, his data tell us that doctors may be able to identify sources of ill health less often than we would like, and when that is the case, we should rely more heavily on the body's own healing mechanisms.

The placebo effect illustrates the power that the content of our thoughts has over the physical processes of our bodies. The effect is so strong that many expensive antidepressants now on the market wouldn't pass trials in which the drug was put up against a sugar pill. Patients have such faith in drugs' effectiveness that their power of belief is as effective as the drug itself. Half of all medications that fail to pass the final trials required by the Food and Drug Administration do so because their effects aren't significantly better than those of fake ones.[23] The trouble isn't that these drugs are ineffective but rather that our powers of belief can be so tremendous that it is hard to separate the body's healing ability from that of the medication.

Benson's relaxation response stimulates the parasympathetic nervous system, or the quiescent system that Andrew Newberg found to be activated in profound spiritual experiences. While he and others have been unable to confirm the effects of intercessory prayer, Benson's research has found that patients with high blood pressure (an average of 146/93.5) could reduce their hypertension by meditation (down to 137/88.9). In some—certainly not all—cases, this reduction allowed patients to return to the normal range and go off medication. The effects remained for as long as the patients meditated. Other studies found that meditation was also related to decreased drug and cigarette use.[24]

Prayer and other religious practices are associated with decreased rates of depression as well. Of ninety-three studies conducted before 2000, a majority showed that stronger religious beliefs and more frequent religious practices seem to reduce the number of people who experienced depression. While the effect is powerful and significant, it's no instant cure.[25] And as with the Cambodian fisherman, religion can be associated with healthful practices without necessarily directly causing better health. In other words, going to church doesn't end depression, but things associated with church, such as having friends who will bring over meals, clean up the house and watch the kids, can help in the treatment of depression.

Depression and other forms of psychological stress have a powerfully negative impact on health by harming the immune system. A lowered sense of well-being reduces the activity of the body's natural killer cells, which protect the body from outside bacteria, viruses and tumors. Depression impairs a number of other essential activities of the immune system. This is another way that faith can affect health. A believer with depression may be more inclined to feel that life is meaningful—even while suffering the full weight of that illness—and such a belief can provide some resistance to the negative immune-system threats of stress.[26]

Another study looked at the effects of faith among a population particularly at risk for depression. Caregivers of cancer patients contend with a host of highly stressful situations and activities in addition to their bereavement due to the impending loss of their loved one. In a study of family caregivers for 175 patients who had died, researchers found that thirteen months later, those who were religious were 26 percent less likely than the nonreligious to have developed major depression.[27]

Practicing our faith gives us the power to pray ourselves into a happier state. This doesn't mean that Christians need be perpetually cheerful; there certainly are other factors in feeling happy. For example, here in the cloudy, rainy climate of the Pacific Northwest, a regular dose of vitamin D during the long, dark winter may provide an even bigger boost to one's mood. I know this from firsthand experience! However, this research does suggest that an ongoing and deepening relationship with God may raise the baseline sense of joy, pleasure and meaningfulness we get out of life. It may not turn a brooding, pensive teenager into a bubbly social butterfly, but it can reverse some of the effects of depression, prompting a person to meet a friend for coffee instead of spending the day in bed.

Spirituality improves health through a number of pathways, among them decreasing depression and increasing social relationships. But spirituality alone can also have a significantly positive impact on the immune system. In a study of people who contracted HIV, researchers found that an increase in spirituality after diagnosis was the most powerful predictor of a patient's viral load (a measure of the extent of the virus's progression) and CD4 cells (agents of the immune system), two measures of the progression of the disease. "Results were independent of church attendance and initial disease status, medication use at every time point, age, gender, race, education, health behaviors, depression, hopelessness, optimism coping, and social support." Another, but weaker, predictor was attendance at religious services.[28]

Wonder-Working Power

For centuries, Christians claimed that the proof of their faith was not only in the logical arguments offered against the pagan philosophers of Greece. While theologians debated the professors of philosophy, many Christians went out to display the truth and the power of the faith through their actions. Just as Jesus healed, so did his disciples, and in the following centuries bishops, missionaries, monks and others all "performed marvelous miracles like Elijah the Tishbite," according to the seventh-century bishop of Amida, in modern Turkey.[29]

These miracles were acknowledged as a significant means by which the early church so quickly spread. Centuries later, Christian apologists, arguing against their Muslim occupiers, disputed the idea that Christianity made rational sense. In the ninth century one old Christian monk in Egypt argued to a Muslim ruler that it is only by miracles that Christianity could have established itself. He said, "I find the proof of the truth of Christianity in its contradictions and inconsistencies which are rejected by intelligence and repelled by the mind because of their difference and contrast."

Instead, the Egyptian monk told his Muslim audience that believers "do not accept or practice [Christianity] except for proofs which they have witnessed, signs which they have known, and miracles which they have recognized, which compelled them to submit to it and practice it." Another Christian philosopher concurred: "The acceptance by those who received [the faith] must have been because of the witness of what the missionaries did in the way of signs opposed to human nature."[30]

Today the working of wonders—whether by drawing out the body's own resources or by divine intervention—remains a primary means by which the Christian faith is growing. Around the world, it is those who experience healing who are quickly becoming Christians. In this consideration of faith and health I would be amiss to avoid this topic, sometimes fraught with controversy. Faith reduces stress, provides people with social support and gives them a sense of meaning. All this affects a person's health and can be measured and tested by researchers. But for most of Christian history, believers have asserted God's personal intervention—in addition to professional medical care—as a potent avenue for healing people in ways outside of typical human experience and immeasurable by science.

Divine Healing

Many believe Pentecostalism to be the fastest-growing religious movement in the world. Along with speaking in tongues, miraculous healing has been a prime feature of Pentecostalism since its beginning. In fact, more Pentecostal Christians claim to have experienced miraculous healing than claim to have spoken in tongues or experienced prosperity.

One study found that fewer than half of Brazilian Pentecostals had spoken in tongues, yet most claimed to have received divine healing. In southern India, researchers have found the same phenomenon: it is healing, not tongues and not prosperity teaching, that attracts people to the church. In China, researchers found that between 80 and 90 percent of converts to Protestant churches joined the church because they or a family member experienced divine healing.[31] There Christians face serious hardship and must make material sacrifices to practice their faith, so it is not prosperity teaching that draws Chinese people to become Christians. Yet healing is commonly expected and experienced.[32]

Across the globe, researchers are finding that in places where the church is rapidly growing, often in less-developed countries with minimal or no access to health care services, the Pentecostal church "makes healing a fundamental element of the gospel, but places almost no emphasis on financial prosperity."[33] On that point, at least, modern Pentecostals and the ancient Egyptian monk would agree.

Still, modern research and history both suggest that Christians have predominantly believed in seeking healing through traditional medicine. "Christians of the first five centuries held views regarding the use of medicine and the healing of disease that did not differ appreciably from those that were widely taken for granted in the Graeco-Roman world," writes historian Gary Ferngren.[34] In fact, Christians had a major role in creating the practice of medicine as we now know it. They believed and taught that God acted "miraculously" on occasion as well, but Christians—especially those who work in medicine—have been realists when it comes to health care miracles. No one since Elijah, not even Jesus, has escaped death.

One of the most studious attempts to get a sense of miraculous healing has been going on for a century. In 1858 in Lourdes, France, a number of people claimed to see the Virgin Mary and to be healed from illness. Since then the site has been a place of pilgrimage for people looking to be healed. Fifty years later, so many people had claimed healing that Pope Pius X declared that the miracles should be investigated. Today the Lourdes Medical Bureau, run strictly by doctors and open to membership of non-Christians, investigates any claim of a miracle. Of the 200 million people who have visited the site, the bureau has declared just sixty-eight miraculous healings, without scientific explanation.[35] As of this writing, only two have occurred since 2000.[36]

If we are to embrace God's omnipotence and omniscience, we cannot discount the ways in which his hand may move beyond human comprehension. Miracles happen. Yet we must hold this knowledge in tension—as best we can—with the reality of creation's utter brokenness. We have seen the ways in which the curse has touched us, down to our very cells, and we have considered how our faith can radically shape our lives. We must not depend on miracles to sustain our faith, yet we cannot demystify the powerful work of God. In the end, whether through the working of a miracle or any the other positive ways our faith affects our health, we can place our hope in Christ. Ultimately, our hope is not in this life but in *new* life in him.

The Doc Who Asks "How Is Your Life Going?"

After sitting on an airplane for twenty-four hours en route to Africa, my knees jammed against the seat in front of me, I began feeling a growing pain in my knees. When I returned home, I sought medical help, but after three doctors in two years, the only things that offered relief were large, clunky braces over both knees. In my summer shorts, I looked like a cyborg in my big black braces.

At a routine physical, I asked my doctor if she would recommend any specialist for my knee pain. She sent me to Kevin Russeau, a chiropractor in Wheaton, Illinois. On my first visit, we chatted casually and he asked not just about my knees but about *me.* He wanted to know about my life. He quickly diagnosed my knee trouble as a result of tight muscles pulling my kneecap out of alignment. He prescribed some exercises, some stretches and a kind of self-massage in which I awkwardly rolled my body over a foam cylinder. Massaging out those knots relaxed the muscles, lengthened them and prevented them from yanking my kneecap out of alignment. After nearly two years of knee pain and lots of requests for prayer, just two weeks of massaging healed them.

During the course of my therapy with Dr. Russeau, I learned that his interest in me, not just my knees, resulted from routinely connecting patients' health to their overall perspective on life. Our visits included questions about the books I brought to read in the waiting room, my job, my writing, my family. More significant, he saw that faith and religious practices had a huge effect on whether or not someone healed.

"The first thing I ask when I see a new patient," Russeau told me, "is 'How is your life going?' The majority of women I ask cry." Usually they have been in a spiral of pain leading to decreased activities, lower quality of life, depression and then more pain. At this point, the pain has usually taken on a life of its own, separate from the original injury. Chronic pain is a learned response. The nerve signals have fired so repeatedly and for so long that the sense of pain is no longer related to the original injury. "You perceive pain in your head," Russeau says. "Your brain interprets that signal, and the emotional centers of the brain interplay with those areas feeling pain."

Belief can be for good or bad, and if we think chronic pain will persist or get worse, it very well may. Over time pain can lead to depression, which reinforces the pain. "I can predict fairly certainly that a patient in this situation won't get rid of their symptoms until they get rid of these other factors," Russeau says. Instead of simply prescribing medication or physical therapy for these patients, he encourages adding some time with a psychologist who might even prescribe meditation.

Russeau says he has seen people dramatically turn their lives around by treating both the physical source of pain and the brain pathways that can threaten to make the pain permanent. Russeau's clinic is a secular one, so when he asks a patient to consider meditation to overcome pain, he often prescribes a form of meditation without any religious content. However, he says, "if an individual has a spiritual life, and if they integrate it into their meditation, it's an even better outcome."

Having a relationship with God, practicing to deepen that relationship and joining others in that practice are all powerful factors in better health. We are subject to all of the brokenness of the fall. But our bodies were designed for more, and as we integrate our faith with our health we catch glimpses of what this deep communion with God and others can look like. Whether we experience miraculous healing, respite from chronic pain or simply the good health that improved relationships can bring, we are experiencing the joys of living out God's design for us.

GOING PUBLIC WITH THE GOOD LIFE

EVERY SUNDAY NIGHT A GROUP GATHERS in our home for worship and a simple soup dinner. We are a lively bunch, children outnumbering adults, but after a few moments of quiet settling, we enter into worship together, spending an hour in prayer while the crockpot full of soup warms on the counter. We pray through the Book of Common Prayer's compline service, an evening prayer service intended to provide closure to the day. We read Scripture, and a skilled musician—a former Air Force Band piano player—leads singing on a guitar. We pray for challenges at work, logistics around a move, family health concerns.

To my surprise, the children in our group love to participate. They offer prayers for friends at school or church and find great joy in being included as readers of passages from Scripture. Because we aren't going through a Bible study or small group curriculum, children can easily participate, even those who can't read. They memorize portions of our prayers and help to lead them; they pass out Bibles to those who need them. They have a deep sense of belonging and participation in the group.

We end our evening with soup and bread and conversation. We

provide soup, friends bring bread, and together we create a fellowship meal. Over time these conversations are knitting us together. Our shared prayer makes conversation flow more freely at the supper table, while our conversation allows our prayer to have a greater resonance because we know the person making the request fairly well. The whole is more than the sum of its parts. The food and conversation combined with the prayer and singing and Scripture add up to an experience that is warm, uplifting and spiritually encouraging.

It is one thing to learn about how prayer stimulates the anterior cingulate, which strengthens our capacity for social relationships and compassion. It is something entirely different to experience it every week. When our daughter described Sunday nights as "a house full of kids and people loving God," I knew we had struck upon something wonderful. There is nothing unique or special about our prayer group. We are simply doing what God designed us for.

Religion Without Faith

Depending on your spiritual disposition, it is possible to look at the research presented in this book and draw conclusions different from those I have drawn. Many researchers see unguided naturalistic evolution shaping humanity over hundreds of thousands of years. They might assume that the trends observed here were bound to happen, given enough time. To them this research is no proof of God, and it certainly isn't proof of God's desire and design for humans to interact with one another and with him.

Evolutionary psychologists argue that religion has been an important and beneficial part of human history, though for social reasons, not spiritual ones. Jonathan Haidt, the New York University cognitive psychologist and author, summarizes this theory. Eons ago humans developed beliefs to explain a world they didn't fully understand. In response to those beliefs came certain practices, like rituals and morals, and those developed into what we now know as religion. These practices tended to help the groups, fostering cooperation—especially moral communities—and explanations of the world that allowed them to survive.

Haidt says that "there is now a great deal of evidence" that religion helps groups succeed.[1] He refers to a study of nineteenth-century communes, which found that twenty years after their founding, only 6 percent of secular communes survived, while 39 percent of religious ones did. Not only that, but the study looked further to see what it was about religion that caused such success. There was "one master variable: the number of costly sacrifices that each commune demanded from its members. . . . The more sacrifice a commune demanded, the longer it lasted." But that was true only of religious communities. The secular ones nearly all failed within eight years, no matter what sacrifices they asked for.[2] Placing extreme demands on people can also be harmful, of course, especially when religious legalism is at work. However, the evidence shows that we human beings do well when we are in a community that loves and cares for its members *while also* guiding behaviors and norms.

"If you live in a religious community," Haidt writes, "you are enmeshed in a set of norms, relationships and institutions that work primarily on the elephant [your subconscious intuitions and inclinations] to influence your behavior. . . . We evolved to live, trade, and trust within shared moral matrices. When societies lose their grip on individuals, allowing all to do as they please, the result is often a decrease in happiness and an increase in suicide."

Haidt argues from a secular liberal standpoint (he doesn't admit to any personal faith in his book) for respecting the contribution religion makes in society, and he isn't alone. Even avowed atheists are trying to create religion without faith. They recognize that religion offers much to appreciate and much that the human spirit needs.

Perhaps the greatest proponent of "religion for atheists" is Alain de Botton, a British philosopher and author of a book by that name. Growing up the son of Jewish atheists, de Botton says that he had no exposure to religion except for his parents' ridicule of it. Yet upon making his own way in the world, he discovered that religious art, music, architecture and community were incredibly attractive. In an interview he says, "That's where my, as I say, crisis of faithlessness came about. I began to realize that religion, for all its flaws and for all its faults and all its excesses, had some high points that were incredibly interesting, fascinating, beautiful, inspiring."[3]

De Botton wants to recapture the communal spirit that faith fosters. We all want goodness and kindness, he says, but we aren't good at actually following through. He says that religions "recognize that we need to have constant public reminders of all this stuff about being good and kind." The religion de Botton seeks to create builds community, teaches values and fosters the best of the human spirit, but he cannot bring himself to include God in the mix.

The long-term success of de Botton's and Haidt's conceptions remains to be seen. But their positions suggest that people are hungry for what faith can offer. They are hungry even for religion, because modern secular society cannot make us delight in those things that lead to a good life. It cannot make us grateful or self-giving. It cannot help us to love or to know that we are loved. And these are the things that lead to human flourishing.

Ears to Hear

For those who have ears to hear, the strong coherence between the ancient wisdom of faith and modern research can be inspiring. God has created not only a biology that allows us to communicate with him in prayer and worship but also a biology to pursue him through spiritual practices, to connect to other people, to love our neighbors as ourselves and to reach out in compassion to those who are suffering. These actions aid (though they don't cure) our physical health, our mental well-being and our sense of living with meaning. And they provide a biological basis for fulfilling the two great commandments to love God with all our heart, mind and strength and to love our neighbors as ourselves. While we need not use modern science as a proof for our faith, it should encourage us to learn that the latest research affirms the ancient words of Jesus, Paul or Augustine.

For many scientists and writers probing these latest discoveries, one of the main lessons of cognitive science is that humans are not rational creatures who choose what is in their own best interest. Instead we seem to be driven by processes below the level of consciousness, processes that we never fully understand and that often conflict with what we want or what we wish we wanted.

Centuries earlier, Augustine of Hippo, the theologian who did the most to set the trajectory of Western Christian thinking, intuitively knew this truth: "Who can map out the various forces at play in one soul, the different kinds of love . . . ? Man is a great depth, O Lord; You number his hairs . . . but the hairs of his head are easier by far to count than his feelings, the movements of his heart."[4] Modern science proves Augustine right. It describes a brain with more possible states than there are particles in the universe, one that we cannot fully know, with too many "forces at play" to comprehend. It describes a brain that produces consciousness not through an executive function but through the welling up of bodily states and a host of brain processes.

What the scientists recognize, however, is that we can shape our behaviors by changing how we think, placing ourselves in a context and with people that support that change, and taking small progressive steps in a new direction.

This wisdom about Christian living fills the Epistles. The apostle Paul expressed it when he wrote that we don't do the good we wish we would do, and instead we do the evil we hate (Rom 7:14-20). He encourages us to offer our bodies as a living sacrifice and be transformed by the renewing of our minds (Rom 12:1-2). Science shows we can indeed become people who do the good we would like to do by shaping the habits of our bodies and even the cells of our brains.

Science is showing that it is not our successes and achievements, our income and wealth, our status in life that make us happy. Instead happiness is about finding meaning in the web of our social networks, caring for other people and putting their needs first, enhancing our compassion, and living within a matrix of beliefs and purpose shared and supported by others. The well-lived life is one in which we lose our life in order to find it. Happiness and joy come from pursuing the good of others rather than our own desires.

Our faith teaches us to knit ourselves into the community of faith. We learn that we are members of a body, the body of Christ, that we have gifts and abilities to contribute but that we also depend on others. We are not individuals separate from one another. In the same way that the hand cannot say to the foot, "I don't need you," we cannot expect to live our spiritual lives with any success in isolation. Our connection to God is integrally woven together with our connections to the people we choose to love.

The Frustrated Path to Goodness

Science and faith seem to agree on what leads to a good life, yet so many aspects of modern life—which science is supposed to have shaped and to keep improving—are opposed to living one. Science can explain very well what a good life is. It can even tell us the kinds of things people who live a good life do, but it cannot help us live one. Science cannot put us into a community; it cannot inspire the emotions that make us desire to live well. Science can empty prayer of its content and meaning and then call it therapy. It can recommend a technique, but it cannot create purpose and goodness. Science describes our world, which allows us to shape it in ways that make our lives easier, even more enjoyable. But it does not provide meaning or joy or purpose or goodness.

This leaves a tremendous gap, because while our culture has embraced science as a path toward better living, at its best science can merely *describe* a good life. Our culture itself is not much help either. Each person is left to determine his or her own course to a good life, and our culture would imply that whatever path we choose might lead us there. However, on our own we tend to do a very bad job at picking a path to a good life. Our best, happiest, most fulfilling lives are possible only when we submit to what is greater than ourselves within the context of supportive relationships in community pursuing the same goal.

This is where the church stands as a beacon to the world, offering a tried and true path toward ultimate fulfillment. Where people are burned by our culture's excessive individualism, by the pursuit of self-fulfillment without any guidance, by the absence of true intimate relationships, by attempts to be spiritual without God or churches and institutions to walk them down the path, they can find in the church something that works.

Sociologist of religion Rodney Stark points to the astounding growth of the early church and says that during times of crisis "Christianity not only seemed to be, but actually was *efficacious*." Stark continues, "At a time when all other faiths were called to question, Christianity offered explanation and comfort. Even more important, Christian doctrine provided a prescription for action. That is, the Christian way appeared to work."[5]

If our exploration of the intersection between spirituality and science is to give us anything, it should confirm the things we have known in our spirits long before now: The Christian way heals, provides meaning, gives hope and offers a path to a good life by connecting us to God and other people. The fingerprints of our loving Creator are evident in our bodies, and our desires for connection and communion are not simply physical necessities but gifts from a God who desires our company.

We may often feel at odds with our culture, but these feelings come from a place deeper than cultural hot-button issues. More profoundly it is because the Christian way of life—deeply connected to others and to God—is easily frustrated by modern life. But that very disconnect illustrates that our society is in need of personal connection to other people and spiritual significance. And perhaps once again Christianity can offer explanation, comfort and a prescription for action.

An Abbey of Unbelievers

Just north of Portland, Oregon, a group of Christians is working to live out their connections to God and one another in very tangible ways. They illustrate beautifully how our body's design to commune with others and with God can lead people to know God by experiencing the love and concern of others.

David Knudtson grew up Pentecostal and met his wife at a Calvary Chapel Bible study. In his twenties the couple became involved in the Vineyard movement through its leader John Wimber. He was a church planter and career pastor until the mid-nineties, when he became involved in the emerging church movement. He had grown dissatisfied with the corporate approach to running a church, so he joined the leadership of an emerging Portland congregation and became a real-estate agent.

David saw the need, in a place like Portland, to stretch the ways in which it was acceptable to be Christian. He wanted to reach out to folks sporting tattoos, piercings and blue hair. David was also drawn to a focus on the poor, the marginalized and those turned off by typical manifestations of the faith.

Eventually he started a church in a bar in Vancouver, just a few miles outside of Portland. When he tried to reproduce the ideas that had worked in Portland, though, the concept fell flat. "This was not what God was doing," he says. "We aren't that hip and cool." It's true, David's typical middle-aged look and goofy joviality are a far cry from Portland's youthful alternative vibe. But God had a different plan for David and his team. "Through my ineptness, God took those things I naturally like, real estate and helping the poor and mentoring young people," he says.

In his real-estate business, David saw that young people were often sharing living space because housing costs were so high. "Let's take that model, refine it and do something for the kingdom," he decided. Meanwhile David's theological journey was taking him away from his Pentecostal upbringing and emerging church experience and toward the more ancient liturgical practices of Anglicanism. There he found a model for a religious community that served the needs of neighbors, which could be adapted to a modern urban setting. He found a way to foster deep connections between people in a way that could lead to deep connections to God.

Arnada Abbey is nothing like anyone's image of an abbey. It isn't a monastic community in any traditional sense. After all, its abbot is a real-estate agent. The abbey's services are held in the living room of a house near downtown Vancouver, Washington, and the house is full of people from the community who are in need of transitional housing.

When I visited Arnada Abbey, about twenty people worshiped in the open living room of a century-old home. In the back were folding tables and chairs, a coffee pot, hot water and tea. People walked in and out freely. Toward the front of the house, large windows had painted crosses on them, sacred music played on a computer, and a small altar stood. A young family, an older couple and several single adults took part in a traditional, though very informal, Anglican service. No one would describe Arnada Abbey as being either hip or high church.

Though the house is used for regular Sunday services, the Abbey rents out its seven rooms to people who need inexpensive housing. David says the Abbey has rules about things like overnight visitors, smoking and taking care of common areas. Anyone who lives there is invited to join in the Abbey's services. Many renters eventually turn to David for counseling or spiritual advice. They bring friends who also turn to the community in times of crisis. "Everyone is welcome to participate, and by definition they are signing up for me to be their spiritual director." David says that of the seven current renters, two have become Christians and three are occasional attendees at services. This is no small feat within the Northwest's nearly pagan culture; it speaks to the spiritual power of connecting to others.

Because of the Abbey's rules, not everyone that David and his wife befriend is ready to live there. So they started a second house where people could also live cheaply but could set up their own rules. "We don't expect non-Christians to live up to our behavior standards," David says. "But we want to be their friend. Maybe later we will be able to lead them to Christ."

The Arnada Abbey is small, but it offers an intimate connection between people, particularly those facing significant needs. "Our ministry on the margins," David says, "isn't anything new but is what the church has always done. It is all about coming into an area, learning, finding needs and meeting needs. That's what God always seems to do."

The stories David tells are of helping someone through an addiction or a broken relationship. He tells of a couple living together who become Christians and get married. In the Pacific Northwest, where hostility to Christianity is very real, Arnada Abbey is practicing a deeply personal way of meeting basic needs as a way to introduce people to God.

Arnada Abbey doesn't have a strategic plan that directs its success. It works simply because this is how God made each one of us. We are designed such that our experience of God and our relationships to other people are bound together. We are made to care for and love one another and to reach out to the Creator himself. Even in a place where people claim to reject God, this kind of practical love opens up a response to connect with God. And as we connect to God, we grow in our ability to connect to other people and respond to their needs with compassion.

What We Were Made For

Whether we find deep connections in time alone in the desert, serving food to others, a soup and prayer group, or more typical church small groups, potlucks or other activities that foster spiritual community, it doesn't take much to look around our lives and pay attention to how we are investing in other people and spiritual practices. Healthy and meaningful lives are built on cups of coffee with friends, helping a neighbor find a place to live, private prayer and worshiping with people we have grown to care for.

Our physical bodies, down to the wiring in our brains and the genes in our cells and the chemicals filling the synapse between neurons, need this kind of faith. We have been designed for it. We are made to perceive and connect to God in a way that changes our very nature. And these changes are made most manifest in the tangible ways that we care for one another. As we connect with God and invite others to join this life of prayer, worship, community and service, we align our biological and spiritual selves with the Creator of the universe and the most fundamental guide for life—loving God and loving others.

ACKNOWLEDGMENTS

I AM IMMENSELY GRATEFUL to the many people who have helped to make this book possible and much better than what I could have on my own. My wife, Clarissa, improved a number of drafts and listened as I talked through ideas while helping me clarify them. She allowed me to slip away in the darkness morning after morning to work on this project. Laura Dailey also helped edit several chapters.

For the last three years I have enjoyed learning a great deal from Brian Sytsma and Rich Stearns at World Vision. I deeply appreciate Brian and Rich's personal support during my wife's illness.

Al Hsu also worked to improve this book, while Ruth Goring did yeoman's work cleaning up the manuscript. I'm incredibly thankful to have been able to work with them and the rest of the IVP staff once more.

NOTES

Introduction: Created for Communion

[1]Andrew Newberg and Mark Robert Waldman, *How God Changes Your Brain: Breakthrough Findings from a Leading Neuroscientist* (New York: Ballantine Books, 2010), pp. 26, 27.

[2]Patrick McNamara, quoted in Barbara Bradley Hagerty, *Fingerprints of God: The Search for the Science of Spirituality* (New York: Riverhead Books, 2009), p. 101.

Chapter 1: Prayer—This Is Your Brain on God

[1]Andrew Newberg and Mark Robert Waldman, *How God Changes Your Brain: Breakthrough Findings from a Leading Neuroscientist* (New York: Ballantine Books, 2010), p. 4.

[2]Andrew Newberg, Eugene d'Aquili and Vince Rause, *Why God Won't Go Away: Brain Science and the Biology of Belief* (New York: Ballantine Books, 2001), pp. 86-90.

[3]Newberg and Waldman, *How God Changes Your Brain*, p. 75.

[4]Ibid., p. 43.

[5]Ibid.

[6]Ibid., pp. 124-26.

[7]Barbara Bradley Hagerty, *Fingerprints of God: The Search for the Science of Spirituality* (New York: Riverhead Books, 2009), p. 118.

[8]Mario Beauregard and Vincent Paquette, "Neural Correlates of a Mystical Experience in Carmelite Nuns," *Neuroscience Letters* 405 (2006): 186-90, www.pucrs.br/feecultura/2010/neural-mysticism.pdf.

[9]Ibid., pp. 274-75.

[10]Newberg and Waldman, *How God Changes Your Brain*, pp. 6-7.

[11]Ibid., p. 14.

[12]Ibid., pp. 6-7.

[13]Evelyn Underhill, *Practical Mysticism: A Little Book for Normal People* (New York: Cosimo Classics, 2006), p. 49.

[14]Antoine Lutz, Julie Brefczynski-Lewis, Tom Johnstone and Richard J. Davidson, "Regulation of the Neural Circuitry of Emotion by Compassion Meditation: Effects of Meditative Expertise," *PLOS ONE* 3, no. 3: e1897, doi:10.1371/journal.pone.0001897.

[15]Christopher K. Germer and Ronald D. Siegel, eds., *Wisdom and Compassion in Psychotherapy: Deepening Mindfulness in Clinical Practice* (New York: Guilford, 2012).

[16]John H. Walton, *The Lost World of Genesis One: Ancient Cosmology and the Origins Debate* (Downers Grove, IL: InterVarsity Press, 2009), p. 26.

[17]N. T. Wright, "Mind, Spirit, Soul and Body: All for One and One for All; Reflections on Paul's Anthropology in His Complex Contexts," http://ntwrightpage.com/Wright_SCP_MindSpiritSoulBody.htm.

[18]Nicole Dudukovic, "This Is Your Brain . . . On Anti-Drug Campaigns," *Remember the Alamo* blog, *Psychology Today*, May 15, 2008, www.psychologytoday.com/blog/remember-the-alamo/200805/is-your-brainon-anti-drug-campaigns.

Chapter 2: Born Connectors

[1]Justin Barrett, *Born Believers: The Science of Children's Religious Belief* (New York: Free Press, 2012), p. 42.

[2]Ibid., p. 7.

[3]Sofia Cavalletti, *The Religious Potential of the Child: Experiencing Scripture and Liturgy with Young Children,* trans. Patricia M. Coulter and Julie M. Coulter (Chicago: Liturgy Training Publications, 1992), p. 43.

[4]David Eagleman, *Incognito: The Secret Lives of the Brain* (New York: Pantheon Books, 2011), p. 83.

[5]Paul Zak, *The Moral Molecule: The Source of Love and Prosperity* (New York: E. P. Dutton, 2013), p. 68.

[6]Tiffany Field, *Touch* (Cambridge, MA: MIT Press, 2001), p. viii.

[7]Ibid., p. 41.

[8]Dacher Keltner, *Born to Be Good: The Science of a Meaningful Life* (New York: W. W. Norton, 2009), p. 111.

[9]Ibid., p. 110.

[10]Harry Harlow's research is summarized in David Brooks, *The Social Animal: The Hidden Sources of Love, Character, and Achievement*

(New York: Random House, 2011), p. 33.

[11]See www.bucharestearlyinterventionproject.org.

[12]Manabu Makinodan, Kenneth M. Rosen, Susumu Ito and Gabriel Corfas, "A Critical Period for Social Experience—Dependent Oligodendrocyte Maturation and Myelination," *Science* 337 (September 14, 2012): 1357-60, www.sciencemag.org/content/337/6100/1357.abstract.

[13]Catherine Stonehouse and Scottie May, *Listening to Children on the Spiritual Journey: Guidance for Those Who Teach and Nurture* (Grand Rapids: Baker Academic, 2010), p. 40.

[14]Barna Group, "Five Reasons Why Millennials Stay Connected to Church," www.barna.org/barna-update/millennials/635-5-reasons-millennials -stay-connected-to-church#.UsLsO2RDvEk.

[15]Chap Clark and Kara Eckman Powell, *Sticky Faith: Everyday Ideas to Build Lasting Faith in Your Kids* (Grand Rapids: Zondervan, 2011), p. 22.

[16]Barna Group, "Most Twentysomethings Put Christianity on the Shelf Following Spiritually Active Teen Years," www.barna.org/barna-update/ article/16-teensnext-gen/147-most-twentysomethings-put-christianity -on-the-shelf-following-spiritually-active-teen-years#.UsGLimRDvEk.

[17]Clark and Powell, *Sticky Faith,* p. 16.

[18]European Commission, *Eurobarometer: Social Values, Science and Technology,* 2005, http://ec.europa.eu/public_opinion/archives/ebs/ebs_225_ report_en.pdf.

[19]Tom Esslemont, "Spirituality in Estonia—the World's 'Least Religious' Country," *BBC News,* www.bbc.co.uk/news/world-europe-14635021.

[20]European Commission, *Eurobarometer.*

[21]Rodney Stark and Roger Finke, *Acts of Faith,* Kindle ed. (Berkeley: University of California Press, 2000), pp. 62-63.

[22]"'Nones' on the Rise," Pew Research on Religion and Public Life Project, October 9, 2012, www.pewforum.org/unaffiliated/nones-on-the-rise.aspx.

[23]Andrew Newberg and Mark Robert Waldman, *How God Changes Your Brain: Breakthrough Findings from a Leading Neuroscientist* (New York: Ballantine Books, 2010), p. 5.

[24]Roy Hattersley, *The Life of John Wesley: A Brand from the Burning* (New York: Doubleday, 2003), p. 32.

Chapter 3: Monkey See, Monkey Do

[1]Marco Iacoboni, *Mirroring People: The New Science of How We Connect*

with Others (New York: Farrar, Straus and Giroux, 2008), p. 34.

[2]Ibid.

[3]Ibid., p. 111.

[4]Ibid., pp. 113-14.

[5]R. B. Zajonc, Pamela K. Adelmann, Sheila T. Murphy and Paula M. Niedenthal, "Convergence in the Physical Appearance of Spouses," *Motivation and Emotion* 11, no. 4 (1987).

[6]Iacoboni, *Mirroring People*, p. 69.

[7]Antonio Damasio, *Descartes' Error: Emotion, Reason, and the Human Brain* (New York: Avon Books, 1994), p. 193.

Chapter 4: Life Together

[1]John Wesley, quoted in Theodore Runyon, "Holiness as the Renewal of the Image of God in the Individual and Society," in *Embodied Holiness: Toward a Corporate Theology of Spiritual Growth*, ed. Samuel Powell and Michael Lodahl (Downers Grove, IL: InterVarsity Press, 1999), p. 81.

[2]Ibid.

[3]Ibid. p. 82.

[4]Gregory Schneider, "Focus on the Frontier Family," *Christian History* 45 (January 1995), www.christianitytoday.com/ch/1995/issue45/4538 .html?start=2.

[5]Malcolm Gladwell, "The Cellular Church: How Rick Warren's Congregation Grew," *New Yorker*, September 12, 2005, www.newyorker.com/ archive/2005/09/12/050912fa_fact_gladwell.

[6]Malcom Gladwell, "The Cellular Church," http://gladwell.com/the -cellular-church/.

[7]Reid Mihalko, quoted in Libby Copeland, "Cuddling and the Self-Taught Sex Coach," *Seattle Times*, September 5, 2004 (originally published in the *Washington Post*), http://seattletimes.com/html/living/2002025448_ cuddleside05.html.

[8]Nicholas Bakalar, "Five-Second Touch Can Convey Specific Emotion, Study Finds," *New York Times*, August 10, 2009, www.nytimes .com/2009/08/11/science/11touch.html?_r=0.

[9]M. J. Hertenstein et al., "Touch Communicates Distinct Emotions," *Emotion* 6, no. 3 (August 2006): 528-33, www.ncbi.nlm.nih.gov/pubmed /16938094.

[10]Jeremy Dean, "Ten Psychological Effects of Nonsexual Touch," *PsyBlog*, April 13, 2011, www.spring.org.uk/2011/04/10-psychological-effects-of -nonsexual-touch.php.

[11]Louis Cozolino, *The Neuroscience of Human Relationships: Attachment and the Developing Social Brain* (New York: W. W. Norton, 2006).

[12]Nicholas A. Christakis and James H. Fowler, *Connected: The Surprising Power of Our Social Networks and How They Shape Our Lives* (New York: Little, Brown, 2009), p. 233.

[13]Ibid.

[14]David Brooks, *The Social Animal: The Hidden Sources of Love, Character, and Achievement* (New York: Random House, 2011), p. 210.

[15]Ibid.

[16]Christakis and Fowler, *Connected,* p. 39.

[17]Beth Azar, "Your Brain on Culture," *Monitor* (APA) 41, no. 10 (November 2010), www.apa.org/monitor/2010/11/neuroscience.aspx.

[18]David Eagleman, *Incognito: The Secret Lives of the Brain* (New York: Pantheon Books, 2011), p. 184.

[19]Christakis and Fowler, *Connected,* pp. 240-43.

[20]Ibid., p. 247.

[21]Ibid., p. 80.

[22]Ibid., p. 51.

[23]Brian Uzzi and Jarrett Spiro, "Collaboration and Creativity: The Small World Problem," *American Journal of Sociology* 111, no. 2 (September 2005), www.kellogg.northwestern.edu/faculty/uzzi/ftp/uzzi's_research_ papers/uzzi&spiroajs_smallworlds.pdf.

[24]Rodney Stark and Roger Finke, "Proposition 52: The Larger the Congregation, the Less Dense the Social Networks Within the Group," in *Acts of Faith,* Kindle ed. (Berkeley: University of California Press, 2000), p. 161.

[25]Ibid., pp. 250-51.

[26]Rick Richardson, *Reimagining Evangelism: Inviting Friends on a Spiritual Journey* (Downers Grove, IL: InterVarsity Press, 2006), p. 27.

[27]Rodney Stark, *The Triumph of Christianity: How the Jesus Movement Became the World's Largest Religion* (San Francisco: HarperOne, 2012), p. 68.

[28]Gerald Sittser, *Water from a Deep Well: Christian Spirituality from Early Martyrs to Modern Missionaries* (Downers Grove, IL: InterVarsity Press, 2007), p. 57.

Chapter 5: Wired for Intimacy

[1]Helen Fisher, *Why We Love: The Nature and Chemistry of Romantic Love* (New York: Henry Holt, 2004), p. 52.

[2]David Brooks, *The Social Animal: The Hidden Sources of Love, Character, and Achievement* (New York: Random House, 2011), p. 207.

[3]Ibid., p. 206.

[4]L. J. Young, "The Neural Basis of Pair Bonding in a Monogamous Species: A Model for Understanding the Biological Basis of Human Behavior," in *Offspring: Human Fertility Behavior in Biodemographic Perspective*, ed. K. W. Wachter and R. A. Bulatao for National Research Council Panel for the Workshop on the Biodemography of Fertility and Family Behavior (Washington, DC: National Academies Press, 2003), p. 4.

[5]Dacher Keltner, *Born to Be Good: The Science of a Meaningful Life* (New York: W. W. Norton, 2009), p. 212.

[6]Ibid., p. 213.

[7]Bernard of Clairvaux, "Preaching the Crusade," quoted in *The World's Best Orations: From the Earliest Period to the Present Time*, ed. David J. Brewer, Edward A. Allen and William Schuyler (St. Louis: Ferd P. Kaiser, 1899), 2:432.

[8]Bernard of Clairvaux, quoted in F. C. Happold, *Mysticism: A Study and an Anthology* (New York: Penguin Books, 1990), p. 234.

[9]T. M. Luhrmann, *When God Talks Back: Understanding the American Evangelical Relationship with God* (New York: Alfred A. Knopf, 2012), p. 80.

[10]"Why Does Liberal Iceland Want to Ban Online Pornography?" *Economist*, April 23, 2013, www.economist.com/blogs/economist-explains/2013/04/economist-explains-why-iceland-ban-pornography.

[11]"Online Pornography to Be Blocked by Default, PM Announces," BBC, July 22, 2013, www.bbc.co.uk/news/uk-23401076.

[12]Norman Doidge, *The Brain That Changes Itself: Stories of Personal Triumph from the Frontiers of Brain Science* (New York: Penguin Books, 2007), p. 103.

[13]Ibid., p. 106.

[14]Ibid., p. 108.

[15]Name changed to protect privacy.

[16]Doidge, *Brain That Changes Itself*, p. 98.

[17]Samuel Crossman, "My Song Is Love Unknown" (1664).

Chapter 6: Strength in Weakness

[1]Adapted from Clarissa Moll, "You Are Not Alone," www.youtube.com/watch?v=g51Jy4wg-0A&lish=PL50PQWgvdsDmGtwcsixQkqpz99KHZkUnz&index=13.

[2]David Eagleman, "The Brain on Trial," *Atlantic*, July/August 2011, www.eaglemanlab.net/papers/Eagleman%20Atlantic%20The%20Brain%20on%20Trial.pdf.

[3]David Eagleman, *Incognito: The Secret Lives of the Brain* (New York: Pantheon Books, 2011), pp. 151-53.

[4]Ibid., p. 155.

[5]Francesca Ducci and David Goldman, "Genetic Approaches to Addiction: Genes and Alcohol," *Addiction* 103, no. 9 (September 2008): 1414-28, http://onlinelibrary.wiley.com/doi/10.1111/j.1360-0443.2008.02203.x/abstract;jsessionid=5EFA44131538EE110BD904CA3788EE8F.f04to1.

[6]Augustine, *Confessions* 8.8, www.ccel.org/ccel/augustine/confessions.xi.html.

[7]Nancy Sherman, *The Untold War: Inside the Hearts, Minds, and Souls of Our Soldiers* (New York: W. W. Norton, 2011), p. 91.

[8]Joel B. Green, *Body, Soul, and Human Life: The Nature of Humanity in the Bible* (Grand Rapids: Baker Academic, 2008), p. 90.

[9]Ibid.

[10]Name has been changed for privacy.

[11]J. I. Packer, *Weakness Is the Way* (Wheaton, IL: Crossway, 2014), pp. 15-16.

[12]Christian Wiman, *My Bright Abyss: Meditation of a Modern Believer*, Kindle ed. (New York: Farrar, Straus and Giroux, 2013), loc. 2097.

[13]Packer, *Weakness Is the Way*, pp. 116-17.

[14]Stephen Post and Jill Neimark, *Why Good Things Happen to Good People: The Exciting New Research That Proves the Link Between Doing Good and Living a Longer, Healthier, Happier Life* (New York: Broadway Books; 2007), p. 55.

[15]Dacher Keltner, *Born to Be Good: The Science of a Meaningful Life* (New York: W. W. Norton, 2009), p. 71.

[16]Ed Dobson, *Seeing Through the Fog* (Colorado Springs: David C. Cook, 2013), pp. 43, 47.

[17]Oliver Sacks, *The Man Who Mistook His Wife for a Hat: And Other Clinical Tales* (New York: Touchstone, 1985), p. 6.

[18]Augustine, quoted in Peter Brown, *Augustine of Hippo: A Biography* (Berkeley: University of California Press, 2000), p. 206.

Chapter 7: Practicing the Disciplines

[1]Dallas Willard, "Spiritual Disciplines, Spiritual Formation and the Restoration of the Soul," *Journal of Psychology and Theology* 26, no. 1 (Spring 1998): 101-9, www.dwillard.org/articles/artview.asp?artID=57.

[2]Stanley Hauerwas, "The Sanctified Body: Why Perfection Does Not Require a 'Self,'" in *Embodied Holiness: Toward a Corporate Theology of Spiritual Growth*, ed. Samuel Powell and Michael Lodahl (Downers Grove, IL: InterVarsity Press, 1999), p. 22.

[3]Willard, "Spiritual Disciplines."

[4]Antonio Damasio, *Descartes' Error: Emotion, Reason, and the Human Brain* (New York: Avon Books, 1994), p. 234.

[5]Malcolm Gladwell, *Blink: The Power of Thinking Without Thinking* (New York: Little, Brown, 2007), pp. 8-10.

[6]Damasio, *Descartes' Error*, p. 213.

[7]William James, "What Is an Emotion?" *Mind* 9 (1884): 188-205, http://psychclassics.yorku.ca/James/emotion.htm.

[8]M. Muraven, R. F. Baumeister and D. M. Tice, "Longitudinal Improvement of Self-Regulation Through Practice: Building Self-Control Strength Through Repeated Exercise," *Journal of Social Psychology* 139, no. 4 (August 1999): 446-57, www.ncbi.nlm.nih.gov/pubmed/10457761.

[9]David Eagleman, *Incognito: The Secret Lives of the Brain* (New York: Pantheon Books, 2011), p. 166.

[10]Ibid., pp. 199-200.

[11]G. K. Chesterton, *Orthodoxy* (New York: John Lane, 1908), p. 32.

[12]Jonathan Haidt, *The Righteous Mind: Why Good People Are Divided by Religion and Politics* (New York: Pantheon Books, 2012), pp. 63-82.

[13]David Brooks, *The Social Animal: The Hidden Sources of Love, Character, and Achievement* (New York: Random House, 2011), p. 22.

[14]Timothy D. Wilson, *Strangers to Ourselves: Discovering the Adaptive Unconscious* (Cambridge, MA: Harvard University Press, 2004), p. 212.

Chapter 8: Worship

[1]Andrew Newberg, Eugene d'Aquili and Vince Rause, *Why God Won't Go Away: Brain Science and the Biology of Belief* (New York: Ballantine Books, 2001), p. 85.

[2]James K. A. Smith, *Desiring the Kingdom: Worship, Worldview, and Cultural Formation* (Grand Rapids: Baker Academic, 2009), p. 25.

[3]John Julius Norwich, *A Short History of Byzantium* (New York: Vintage Books, 1997), p. 66.

[4]Alexander Rentel, "Byzantine and Slavic Orthodoxy," in *Oxford History of Christian Worship*, ed. Geoffrey Wainwright and Karen B. Westerfield Tucker (Oxford: Oxford University Press, 2006), pp. 266-67.

[5]Timothy Ware, *The Orthodox Church* (London: Penguin Books, 1997), p. 264.

[6]Rentel, "Byzantine and Slavic Orthodoxy," p. 262.

[7]Ibid., p. 275.

[8]Ibid., p. 291.

[9]Ibid., p. 274.

[10]James K. Wellman Jr., Katie E. Corcoran and Kate Stockly-Meyerdirk, "'God Is Like a Drug . . .': Explaining Interaction Ritual Chains in American Megachurches," www.scribd.com/doc/103623517/UW-Megachurch-Study.

[11]Ibid.

[12]Ibid.

[13]John Medina, *Brain Rules: 12 Principles for Surviving and Thriving at Work, Home, and School* (Seattle: Pear, 2010), pp. 104-5.

Chapter 9: Acts of Service

[1]Diana Garland, *Family Ministry: A Comprehensive Guide* (Downers Grove, IL: InterVarsity Press, 2012), p. 423.

[2]Ibid.

[3]Ibid., p. 424.

[4]Robert D. Putnam and David E. Campbell, *American Grace: How Religion Divides and Unites Us*, Kindle ed. (New York: Simon and Schuster, 2010), loc. 6604-5.

[5]Ibid., loc. 6582-83.

[6]Gerald Huther, *The Compassionate Brain: How Empathy Creates Intelligence*, trans. Michael H. Kohn (Boston: Trumpeter Books, 2006), p. 13.

[7]Dacher Keltner, *Born to Be Good: The Science of a Meaningful Life* (New York: W. W. Norton, 2009), p. 248.

[8]Ibid., p. 249.

[9]Andrew Newberg, Eugene d'Aquili and Vince Rause, *Why God Won't Go*

Away: Brain Science and the Biology of Belief (New York: Ballantine Books, 2001), pp. 124-26.

[10]Ibid.

[11]Ibid.

[12]Keltner, *Born to Be Good*, p. 229.

[13]Ibid., p. 242.

[14]Ibid., p. 230.

[15]"Matthew Emerzian ('97) Makes Every Monday Matter," UCLA Anderson School of Management, August 3, 2012, www.anderson.ucla.edu/media-relations/2012/matthew-emerzian.

[16]Watch Matthew's TED talk at www.youtube.com/watch?v=xAcHpoWBbBQ.

[17]Paul Zak, *The Moral Molecule* (New York: Bantam Books, 2012), p. xi.

[18]Keltner, *Born to Be Good*, p. 13.

[19]Ibid., p. 71.

Chapter 10: Neuro-transformation

[1]Andrew Newberg, Eugene d'Aquili and Vince Rause, *Why God Won't Go Away: Brain Science and the Biology of Belief* (New York: Ballantine Books, 2001), p. 161.

[2]Nicholas Humphrey, *A History of the Mind: Evolution and the Birth of Consciousness* (New York: Springer, 1999), p. 79.

[3]Aislinn Laing, "British Soldier Blinded in Iraq Trials New Technology to 'See' Using His Tongue," *Telegraph*, March 2, 2010, www.telegraph.co.uk/health/healthnews/7350218/British-soldier-blinded-in-Iraq-trials-new-technology-to-see-using-his-tongue.html.

[4]Sandra Blakeslee, "'Rewired' Ferrets Overturn Theories of Brain Growth," *New York Times*, April 25, 2000, www.nytimes.com/2000/04/25/science/rewired-ferrets-overturn-theories-of-brain-growth.html.

[5]Norman Doidge, *The Brain That Changes Itself: Stories of Personal Triumph from the Frontiers of Brain Science* (New York: Penguin Books, 2007), p. 43.

[6]Andrew Newberg and Mark Robert Waldman, *How God Changes Your Brain: Breakthrough Findings from a Leading Neuroscientist* (New York: Ballantine Books, 2010), p. 104.

[7]Ibid., p. 14.

[8]Newberg, d'Aquili and Rause, *Why God Won't Go Away*, p. 161.

[9]Doidge, *Brain That Changes Itself*, pp. 155-56.

[10]Bill Hybels, *Too Busy Not to Pray* (Downers Grove, IL: InterVarsity Press, 2008), p. 11.

Chapter 11: The Great Physician

[1]Herbert Benson et al., "Study of the Therapeutic Effects of Intercessory Prayer (STEP) in Cardiac Bypass Patients: A Multi-center Randomized Trial of Uncertainty and Certainty of Receiving Intercessory Prayer," May 2005, www.templeton.org/pdfs/press_releases/060407STEP_paper.pdf.

[2]Gregory M. Lamb, "Study Highlights Difficulty of Isolating Effect of Prayer on Patients," *USA Today*, April 2, 2006, www.usatoday.com/tech/science/2006-04-02-prayer-study_x.htm (orig. *Christian Science Monitor*).

[3]Benson et al., "Study of the Therapeutic Effects."

[4]Richard Sloan, quoted in Benedict Carey, "Long-Awaited Medical Study Questions the Power of Prayer," *New York Times*, March 31, 2006, www.nytimes.com/2006/03/31/health/31pray.html.

[5]Harold Koenig, quoted in Lamb, "Study Highlights Difficulty."

[6]Candy Gunther Brown, *Testing Prayer: Science and Healing* (Cambridge, MA: Harvard University Press, 2012), p. 91.

[7]Ibid., p. 1.

[8]Ibid.

[9]Andrew Newberg, Eugene d'Aquili and Vince Rause, *Why God Won't Go Away: Brain Science and the Biology of Belief* (New York: Ballantine Books, 2001), p. 130.

[10]Harold Koenig, *Medicine, Religion, and Health: Where Science and Spirituality Meet* (West Conshohocken, PA: Templeton Foundation Press, 2008), p. 22.

[11]Ibid., p. 24.

[12]Tracy Balboni et al., "Support of Cancer Patients' Spiritual Needs and Associations with Medical Care Costs at the End of Life (419-C)," *Journal of Pain and Symptom Management* 41, no. 1 (2011): 243-44.

[13]Koenig, *Medicine, Religion, and Health*, p. 38.

[14]Ibid., pp. 52-53.

[15]Ibid.

[16]Ibid., pp. 56-57.

[17]Ibid., p. 57.

[18]Ibid.

[19]Herbert Benson, *The Relaxation Response* (New York: HarperCollins, 2000), pp. xli-xlii.

[20]Ibid., p. 21.

[21]Herbert Benson and Marg Stark, *Timeless Healing: The Power and Biology of Belief* (New York: Scribner, 1996), pp. 154-55.

[22]Ibid., p. 49.

[23]Steve Silberman, "Placebos Are Getting More Effective. Drugmakers Are Desperate to Know Why," *Wired*, August 24, 2009, available at www.mindpowernews.com/PlacebosStronger.htm.

[24]Benson, *Relaxation Response*, p. 114.

[25]Koenig, *Medicine, Religion, and Health*, p. 69.

[26]Ibid., p. 39.

[27]Ibid., pp. 72-73.

[28]Ibid., p. 87.

[29]Philip Jenkins, *The Lost History of Christianity* (San Francisco: HarperOne, 2009), p. 75.

[30]Ibid., p. 76.

[31]Candy Gunther Brown, "Introduction: Pentecostalism and the Globalization of Illness and Healing," in *Global Pentecostal and Charismatic Healing*, ed. C. G. Brown (New York: Oxford University Press, 2011), p. 14.

[32]See also David Wang and Georgina Sam, *Christian China and the Light of the World: Miraculous Stories from China's Great Awakening* (Ventura, CA: Regal/Gospel Light, 2013).

[33]Brown, "Introduction," p. 14.

[34]Gary Fergren, *Medicine and Health Care in Early Christianity* (Baltimore: Johns Hopkins University Press, 2009), p. 13.

[35]Dan Buckley, "A Doctor, Not a Miracle Worker: Medical Volunteering in Lourdes," *Irish Examiner*, February 22, 2014, www.irishexaminer.com/ireland/a-doctor-not-a-miracle-worker-medical-volunteering-in-lourdes-259608.html.

[36]"Miracles Under the Microscope," *Economist*, April 20, 2000, www.economist.com/node/304212.

Chapter 12: Going Public with the Good Life

[1]Jonathan Haidt, *The Righteous Mind: Why Good People Are Divided by Religion and Politics* (New York: Pantheon Books, 2012), p. 256.

[2]Ibid., p. 257.

[3]Alain de Botton, "A School of Life for Atheists," interview by Krista Tippett, *On Being,* September 6, 2012, www.onbeing.org/program/transcript/4831#main_content.

[4]Peter Brown, *Augustine of Hippo: A Biography* (Berkeley: University of California Press, 2000), p. 166.

[5]Rodney Stark, *The Rise of Christianity: A Sociologist Reconsiders History* (Princeton, NJ: Princeton University Press, 1996), p. 78.

ABOUT THE AUTHOR

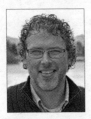

Rob Moll is an award-winning journalist and editor-at-large with *Christianity Today*. He has written extensively on health and health-care issues, investing and personal finance, religion and rural America. His work has appeared in the *Wall Street Journal, Books & Culture* and *Leadership*. He has also served as a hospice volunteer. Rob serves World Vision as communications officer to the president and lives in the Seattle area.

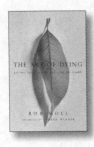

Also by Rob Moll
The Art of Dying
ISBN 978-0-8308-3736-6